Management of
Neurological Disorders

Management of Neurological Disorders

Bryan Ashworth M.D. F.R.C.P.

Consultant Neurologist, Neurological Unit, Northern General Hospital, Edinburgh
Senior Lecturer in Medical Neurology, University of Edinburgh

Michael Saunders M.B. F.R.C.P.

Consultant Neurologist, Northern Regional Health Authority and Newcastle Area Health Authority (Teaching)
Associate Lecturer in Clinical Neurology, University of Newcastle upon Tyne

Foreword by

Professor John N. Walton T.D. M.D. D.Sc. F.R.C.P.

Dean of Medicine and Professor of Neurology, University of Newcastle upon Tyne

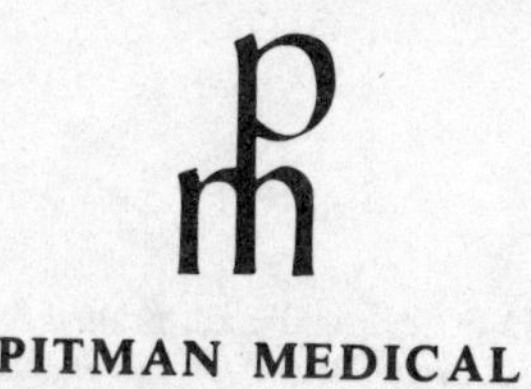

PITMAN MEDICAL

First published 1977

Cat. No. 21 0023 81

Pitman Medical Publishing Co Ltd
42 Camden Road, Tunbridge Wells,
Kent TN1 2QD

Associated Companies

UNITED KINGDOM
Pitman Publishing Ltd, London
Focal Press Ltd, London

USA
Fearon–Pitman Publishers Inc, California

AUSTRALIA
Pitman Publishing Pty Ltd, Melbourne

CANADA
Pitman Publishing, Toronto
Copp Clark Publishing, Toronto

EAST AFRICA
Sir Isaac Pitman and Sons Ltd, Nairobi

SOUTH AFRICA
Pitman Publishing Co SA (Pty) Ltd, Johannesburg

NEW ZEALAND
Pitman Publishing NZ Ltd, Wellington

British Library Cataloguing in Publication Data

Ashworth, Bryan
Management of neurological disorders
1. Nervous system—Diseases
I. Title II. Saunders, Michael
616.8 RC346

ISBN: 0–272–79421–X

Text set in 11/12 pt Photon Times, printed by photolithography
and bound in Great Britain at The Pitman Press, Bath

Contents

	Foreword	vi
	Preface	ix
	Acknowledgements	x
1.	Intensive Care	1
2.	Rehabilitation	14
3.	Psychiatric Aspects of Neurology	24
4.	The Neurogenic Bladder	34
5.	Chronic Pain	43
6.	Headache and Facial Pain	55
7.	Epilepsy	62
8.	Parkinsonism and Involuntary Movement	81
9.	Special Senses	92
10.	Dementia and Degenerative Disorders	103
11.	Multiple Sclerosis	112
12.	Cerebral Vascular Disease	127
13.	Head Injuries	137
14.	Cerebral Tumours	146
15.	Developmental Disorders	158
16.	Spinal Cord Disorders	168
17.	Disorders of the Cranial Nerves and Peripheral Nervous System	180
18.	Motor Neurone Disease, Myasthenia Gravis, and Muscle Disease	199
19.	Infections and Infestations	216
20.	Metabolic Disorders	238
	References	259
	Recommended Reading	260
	Appendixes:	
1.	Voluntary Organisations in the United Kingdom	263
2.	Financial Allowances in the United Kingdom and Other Sources of Help	265
3.	Proprietary Drugs	267
	Index	271

Foreword

by

John N. Walton, T.D., M.D., D.Sc., F.R.C.P.

Dean of Medicine and Professor of Neurology, University of Newcastle upon Tyne

When I was a medical student, and even after I qualified in medicine, the view was widely prevalent that neurological medicine represented a rather cold and intellectual discipline, predominantly concerned with the diagnosis of rare and abstruse disease entities or with the localisation of lesions to a very precise anatomical point in the nervous system. Knowledge of neuroanatomy and of neurophysiology was thought to be the firm basis of neurological practice but neuropharmacology was in its infancy and many joking references were constantly made about 'that specialty in which there is no treatment'. In the last 30 years there have been remarkable advances in the treatment of many neurological disorders, some based upon fundamental pharmacological evidence; the introduction of levodopa for the treatment of Parkinsonism is an excellent example. Advances in management have also been many; we have passed through the era of explosive developments in neuroradiology and brain scanning and are now well launched upon that of computerised transaxial tomography.

These and many other important developments are highlighted in this book by Drs. Ashworth and Saunders. It is not a textbook of neuropharmacology nor a compendium of physical and other methods of treating neurological disease. Rather is this a short manual of practical guidance, written for medical students, house officers and practising physicians, in which the authors share with the reader the fruits of their personal experience and explain how they believe it is best to manage patients with neurological disease. Beginning with chapters on intensive care and rehabilitation, they go on to discuss successively the main presenting features, differential diagnosis, investigation and management of patients suffering from some of the commoner syndromes, symptom-complexes and disease entities seen in clinical practice. The text is succinct, yet I have found it very readable. Not every neurologist or physician will agree with every comment or every piece of advice which the book contains, as brevity, though always commendable, can occasionally lead to dogmatism; and after all, there are still many aspects of treatment in neurology which remain controversial. But I have no doubt that many readers will enjoy reading this short volume and will benefit from the guidance which it offers. A short primer upon the management of neurological disorders was needed and Drs. Ashworth and Saunders have filled an important lacuna in the list of neurological texts now extant by giving us this work.

John N. Walton

Cur'd yesterday of my disease
I died last night of my physician

Matthew Prior 1664–1721

Success in treatment signifies the correct application of all therapeutic measures.

Charaka Samhiti
7th Century B.C.

Preface

Our primary aim in presenting this book is to deal with the management of common neurological disorders as concisely as possible. It is intended as a guide to clinical practice and we hope that it will also be useful to those who are preparing for examinations. A short work of this kind must rest heavily on the writings of others, and while we are very conscious of this we have not attempted a comprehensive bibliography. A list of books for further reading, and specific references to some of the more specialised treatments will be found at the end of the book. Our purpose has been to distil contemporary trends in the light of our own experience as clinical neurologists.

Three themes pervade the book: intensive care, rehabilitation, and drug therapy. A glance at the list of chapter headings will reveal that we have followed a clinical plan and have used groupings that reflect common diseases and disorders. We begin with an outline of intensive care, rehabilitation, the psychiatric aspects of neurology, the neurogenic bladder, and the relief of chronic pain. Then follows a series of chapters on clinical management that can be read separately. The coverage provided in these chapters sometimes goes beyond our day-to-day experience but we have thought it important to consider the physician's view of cerebral tumours and head injuries. An account of the management of developmental disorders has been included. The closing chapters deal with infections and metabolic disorders.

Description of disease has been reduced to a minimum, but it seemed appropriate to mention aetiology and to discuss differential diagnosis in relation to the investigation of the patient. If such investigation is to be purposeful it must be directed to the recognition of conditions that can be treated, rather than the mere collection of data. We have had some difficulty in deciding what to leave out. In general, we have confined ourselves to the strictly neurological aspects of treatment and have deliberately omitted mental retardation, neonatal problems, and paediatric neurology.

In discussing surgical treatment we have avoided operative detail but have tried to convey a picture of what is involved and the results that can be expected in skilled hands.

In summary, the book attempts to show what the neurological services are trying to achieve and how far these aims are currently realised.

M.S.
B.A.

Acknowledgements

We are grateful to Professor John N. Walton for writing the foreword and for his constructive comments. We wish to thank Dr E. B. French for his advice on the management of infections and Dr I. W. B. Grant for help with the section on respiratory intensive care.

Mrs K. E. McGeorge and Miss Christine Oliver have given invaluable help in typing the manuscript and Mr Stephen Neal has encouraged us throughout this venture.

1

Intensive Care

Increasing sophistication of medical treatment has resulted in the development of intensive care units. Under ideal conditions, the same facilities can be provided in a ward or side room, but economy, organisation and training of staff favour the grouping of patients. In the general hospital the proportion of neurological patients who need intensive care is small and is insufficient to justify a unit for their exclusive use. Often they will be accommodated alongside patients with respiratory or cardiac disease.

Selection of Patients. The satisfactory running of a unit requires careful selection of patients. There is no place for the terminal case of chronic disease. It is best confined to the management, over a period of days or weeks, of patients judged to be likely to benefit significantly from the special skills that are applied.

Staff. The work makes great demands on nursing and medical personnel. The nurse has greater responsibility than in an ordinary ward, and will often have to act quickly and initiate a prearranged programme of treatment. The staff must be fully trained and continuously available. The pace of events and the inevitable failures in treatment have an effect on staff morale. It is important that an atmosphere of calm and cheerfulness is created, and this is also a factor in staff selection. The medical management also presents problems, and it must be clear to everyone concerned which consultant is responsible for the management of each patient. The skills of the anaesthetist are often required. The unit can conveniently be administered by a specialist in intensive care, an anaesthetist, or a chest physician. Regular consultation with other experts is essential.

Environment. The environment of the intensive care unit is highly significant, because most patients will have difficulty in concentrating on any activity other than their own treatment for longer than a few minutes. The room should provide adequate space, be well lit, and, if possible, have views that preserve contact with normal activities. It should be quiet and situated away from noisy corridors. Buzzers and flashing lights should be reduced to a minimum.

Observation and Monitoring. Charting of the pulse rate, blood pressure, respiratory rate, core and skin temperature, and fluid balance is usually a routine. The frequency of observations will vary with the case, and computer systems are useful for on-line recording.

Skin temperature is conveniently recorded using a probe, and core temperature with a probe in the external auditory meatus or lower oesophagus. Rectal temperature measurements carry some risk of spread of infection. A continuous display of the cardiograph on an oscilloscope is useful. Central venous pressure can be monitored with a catheter in the right atrium. Chest radiographs must be easily obtained, usually with portable equipment.

These are basic requirements, but the use of computers provides for more elaborate records and automatic alarm signals. Closed circuit television is no substitute for the presence of staff adjacent to the bed.

While these facilities can be expected in a unit, many aspects of intensive care impinge on daily management of patients who do not require all the facilities of the special unit. Some of these will now be considered in a general way to avoid repetitive discussion later in the book. No attempt is made to cover all aspects of the subject, and only points of special significance for the neurological patient will be discussed.

Recognition of Change. The general observation and monitoring of the patient are designed to ensure early recognition of any change in the condition, and particularly any deterioration.

In assessing conscious level, it is best to record the type of response, rather than rely on numerical or other grading which may vary in significance according to different observers. It is useful to record the patient's conscious level in such terms as: alert, responding readily to command, responding to command but tending to lapse into a drowsy state when not stimulated (stupor), responsive to pinch or pin-prick, responsive to supraorbital pressure, or unresponsive. Coma must, of course, be distinguished from sleep, and some people are difficult to rouse from the deep phase of sleep.

Changes in temperature, pulse rate, respiration, and blood pressure must always be noted. A rise of 0·5°C (1°F) in temperature is likely to cause the pulse rate to rise by about 10 beats a minute. A fall in pulse rate may be associated with a rise in intracranial pressure, and is seen particularly in patients with expanding intracranial haematoma. Rise in blood pressure may be attributable to restlessness, distension of the bladder, respiratory distress, a rise in intracranial pressure, or other factors. There is a fall in blood pressure in shock which must alert the observer to the possibility of there being haemorrhage outside the nervous system. It may also be caused by electrolyte disorder (low sodium) or adrenal failure.

Among the neurological signs, the state of the pupils, deviation of the eyes, ptosis, and the development of immobility or flaccidity of a limb are most important. The pupils should not be dilated for the purpose of examining the fundi in detail because this may deprive the observer of valuable pupillary signs for several hours. An adequate view of the optic disc can almost always be obtained by an experienced observer without dilatation of the pupils if the room is darkened. The most significant feature is dilatation of a pupil with loss of response to light.

A generalised convulsion or a focal epileptic attack must always be recorded. The pattern of the attack, and particularly the part first affected, should be noted. After an attack, there may be flaccid weakness (Todd's paralysis) and depression of the conscious level, both of which are temporary. A solitary attack of this kind is not an indication for therapy, and it is important to avoid phenobarbitone and other sedatives likely to complicate the clinical picture. If the fits continue, or status epilepticus develops, further measures are required. Phenytoin 300 mg daily may be given by gastric tube as a prophylactic. When control is more urgent 10 mg of diazepam are given intravenously and followed by an infusion of 100 mg during the next twelve hours. When the patient is already receiving assisted respiration, fits may be controlled with tubocurarine or a similar drug, but if the patient is conscious their effects must be explained to him.

Management of Coma. The first aim in coma is to preserve the normal physiological functions as far as possible, and this is supplemented by measures to deal with its cause.

The *airway* must be kept clear and in patients with chest disease or respiratory failure a tracheostomy may be needed. When this is not required, a simple airway is inserted, and accumulated secretions cleared by suction and by tilting the patient. Comatose patients should not lie supine and must be moved frequently.

Adequate fluid intake must be maintained, usually with a nasogastric tube. A fluid diet and the drug therapy can be given by the same route.

An intravenous drip is needed when the electrolyte balance is disturbed or gastric absorption is not satisfactory, and is also convenient for the administration of drugs. The blood urea, serum sodium, potassium, and bicarbonate must be checked as a matter of urgency. If the patient shows no sign of dehydration and the electrolyte levels are within the reference range, it should be possible to manage the fluid intake and feeding by means of a gastric tube. A high serum sodium may be due to reduced intake of fluid and can be corrected by giving 5 per cent intravenous dextrose. A low serum sodium may be related to vomiting or excessive sweating and will require correction by infusion of sodium chloride injection 150 mmol/litre (0·9 per cent).

A low potassium level may be brought about by massive intravenous infusions of fluid low in potassium, and particularly in a patient deprived of the normal dietary intake. Potassium can be given by gastric tube in the form of effervescent solution or intravenously as potassium chloride. The use of intravenous potassium demands special care. It can be given as dextrose and potassium chloride solution which contains 40 mmol potassium per litre, and the rate of infusion should not exceed 20 mmol/hr. It is seldom necessary to give more than 60 mmol/day.

High serum potassium is found in patients with renal failure and is aggravated by trauma to tissues or tissue breakdown due to other causes. When the level exceeds 6 mmol there is a risk of cardiac arrest. The cardiograph may show T wave tenting followed by irregularities, increase in the R wave, and a biphasic tracing. The serum potassium level may be lowered by intravenous infusion of 5 per cent glucose, and soluble insulin in doses of 20 units.

Bladder drainage must be ensured and an indwelling catheter is usually needed. The urinary output should be maintained above one litre daily.

If the patient is febrile the cause must be ascertained. It is commonly an infection of the urinary tract or chest. Appropriate antibiotic therapy can then be given, but we find no indication for routine antibiotic administration to patients in coma.

The patient in coma must be turned regularly and at least every two hours for only in this way can pressure sores be prevented. If redness appears or ulceration develops, pressure on the affected area must be avoided completely.

The Paralysed Patient. When the limbs are paralysed it is vital that passive movements are carried out daily to prevent contractures and immobilisation of the joints. Light splints help to preserve the position of the limb. When power returns more active exercise can be encouraged.

Problems of Communication. The paralysed or aphasic patient may have great difficulty in making his needs known, but it is usually possible to decide whether the patient with motor aphasia or a tracheostomy can understand speech. Signalling devices and the use of cards with key words may help him to convey messages and answer questions. Various methods are available for turning the pages of a book. An angled rod may be attached to a headband or a mouthstick that has been properly fitted. Electrically operated page turners may be needed for those who are severely disabled.

RESPIRATORY FAILURE

Intensive care directed to the management of respiratory failure is important in some patients with disease of the nervous system. Fortunately, such patients are few, but their proper management may well result in survival when they would otherwise have died. Respiratory intensive care makes great demands on staff and facilities, particularly staff, and it is indicated only in those situations where temporary assistance with breathing may tide the patient over a crisis, and there is potential for recovery. This applies in acute infections such as poliomyelitis and tetanus, acute polyneuropathy, myasthenia gravis, status epilepticus, polymyositis, head injury, and in some cases of drug-induced coma. Respiration can be maintained with relatively simple equipment as a temporary measure. When prolonged care is required the patient should be transferred to a special unit. Intermittent positive pressure respiration is the usual method and has replaced the Drinker type of tank respirator. There is, occasionally, a place for the cuirass equipment.

Assessment of Respiratory Function. Assessment must take account of the nature of the neurological disease, its effects on respiratory control—both central and peripheral—the presence or absence of bulbar involvement, the presence of chronic respiratory disease or chest deformity, the effects of infection or inhalation, and circulatory disturbance.

The first consideration must be to see that the airway is not obstructed. Obstruction due to secretions, food or other foreign material may be cleared by suction and by posturing the patient in the semi-prone position with the head lowered. The jaw is lifted and a gag inserted, if necessary, to control the position of the tongue. The extent of bulbar involvement may be assessed by taking account of any history of dysphagia, ability to protrude the tongue and move it from side to side, and movements of the palate. In the absence of facial weakness, the patient with palatal incompetence will be unable to blow out the cheeks unless the nose is occluded. A useful simple test is to ask the patient to count up to 20 without taking a breath.

Movement of the diaphragm can be assessed clinically by observing the abdomen from one side. When a deep breath is taken the diaphragm descends and causes the abdominal wall to bulge. If there is bilateral diaphragmatic paralysis this movement is not seen and the abdominal wall may retract on inspiration. Unilateral paralysis may not be detected by a clinical assessment. The accessory muscles can be seen to lift the chest wall when respiration is seriously impaired. It is important to determine whether the patient can cough and clear secretions. At the same time a clinical examination of the chest and a radiograph may provide useful information.

Radiographic screening of the diaphragm may be used to detect unilateral paralysis. The patient is asked to sniff; the normal side of the diaphragm descends but the paralysed side rises. Bilateral paralysis is easily overlooked because there may be very little movement and no rise on inspiration.

Respiratory failure can be considered in two stages. In the early phase there is dyspnoea on exertion but ventilation is adequate at rest. Later, ventilatory failure supervenes; it is defined as a state in which the partial pressure of carbon dioxide in arterial blood (PaCO2) is raised above 40 mmHg. Laboratory tests of particular value in the assessment of doubtful cases include the forced expiratory volume in one second (FEV1). When this falls to 800 ml or less the patient is likely to need assisted respiration. Inability to cough may be an indication for assisted respiration even if the FEV1 is greater than 1 litre.

Indications for Intensive Respiratory Care. It is important that assisted respiration is considered for any patient who becomes breathless or has difficulty in coughing. Respiratory intensive care units prefer to observe doubtful cases rather than receive them at the stage of severe hypoxia.

If intensive respiratory care is necessary the manner in which the patient is transported to the special unit is important. Relief of any obstruction of the airway, postural drainage, and the need for intubation of the trachea or, rarely, tracheostomy should be considered before the patient is moved. Oxygen may be useful in a borderline case. In most of the diseases under consideration it is likely that when assisted respiration is required it will have to be continued over a period of days, and it is at this stage that the value of a team accustomed to handling such problems shows itself. As an emergency measure a cuffed endotracheal tube (soft seal cuff) inserted through the mouth or nose under local anaesthesia will ensure a clear airway, and the cuff will prevent secretions descending into the bronchi. When an endotracheal tube is kept in position for more than 72 hours there is increasing risk of damage to the mucosa and ulceration of the trachea or of a main blood vessel, with catastrophic effect. The vocal cords may be injured by prolonged intubation, therefore it is necessary to decide at an early stage whether tracheostomy would be preferable. It is usually indicated when there is weakness of the bulbar muscles.

Technique in Management of Assisted Respiration. The management of respiratory problems of this type requires continuous attendance on the part of the staff. Emergencies due to accumulation of secretions, technical faults in the equipment, power failure, and other hazards may develop. When a satisfactory airway has been established attention will be needed to prevent accumulation of secretions. Intubation or tracheostomy facilitate control of secretions and reduce the dead space. Administered gases must be humidified to prevent drying of secretions. The machine used must be adjusted for pressure applied and the volume of gas exchanged. Various models are available and some are patient-triggered so that the respirator supplements the patient's own breathing. Such equipment must maintain breathing automatically if not triggered. In most cases it is more satisfactory if the patient allows the machine to breathe for him at the rate of about 20 respirations a minute.

Over-inflation may cause the lung to be distended unduly. When the volume exchanged is too great, carbon dioxide will be washed out of the respiratory system causing the patient to adapt to a lower intensity of central respiratory stimulation, which may aggravate the difficulties when the patient is weaned from the respirator.

The importance of reducing pressure on the wall of the trachea has been mentioned; the cuff around the tube must be released at regular intervals. Another hazard with an endotracheal tube is the possibility of inserting it into a bronchus (when the cuff may occlude the other bronchus) and in unskilled hands there is the risk that it may be inserted into the oesophagus. Feeding by a nasal tube is needed when an endotracheal tube is in use; the fluid intake can then be controlled and adequate nutrition provided. The patient with a tracheostomy will manage without a feeding tube if bulbar function is intact, but food and fluid may then exude around the tracheostomy, a feature that should not be confused with the development of a fistula. Intravenous infusion is convenient for administering drugs. The electrocardiograph should be monitored continuously until respiration is controlled to ensure detection of any cardiac arrhythmia. Pulse rate, temperature, and blood pressure should be recorded at hourly intervals. The patient must also be turned frequently to prevent bed sores—particularly if he is paralysed or comatose—and passive movements are necessary to prevent venous thrombosis in the limbs. In cases of infection, sputum culture will guide antibiotic therapy. Daily arterial blood gas analysis is needed as a check. If the power supply fails an emergency generator may be used. Alternatively, the respirator may be controlled manually or an Ambu bag employed. Electric torches must always be available.

When the time comes for the respirator to be withdrawn the effect of disconnecting the machine will first be observed. A good deal of personal attention and reassurance to the patient is needed at this stage. A distinction should be made between voluntary effort to breathe and normal spontaneous respiration. Fatigue is often prominent. Blood gases should be checked after an hour. Weaning from the respirator should always be done during the day.

Management of patients with various neurological diseases.

Acute Poliomyelitis and Polyneuritis. In these conditions respiratory problems may develop rapidly at an early stage of the illness and even at a time when the diagnosis is in doubt. A patient with acute poliomyelitis is most likely to develop acute respiratory failure within 48 hours of the onset of any neurological features (onset of major illness). It may develop due to bulbar involvement, with denervation of the larynx, paralysis of the phrenic nerves or the nerves to intercostal and accessory muscles of respiration. All these mechanisms may be involved but it is characteristic of poliomyelitis that the disease may be patchy in its neurological effects. Respiratory failure in poliomyelitis will usually require control over a period of several weeks at least.

In the acute polyradiculopathy of *Guillain-Barré syndrome* the onset may be rapid. The patient usually develops paraesthesiae and limb weakness which may progress over a period of a few hours or days to dense paralysis and respiratory failure. Sometimes the onset of respiratory failure is less abrupt than this, but in the course of this disorder respiratory failure is most likely in the first fortnight and is seldom delayed beyond the third week. If it does supervene, a period of two to three weeks on the respirator will usually be needed, hence tracheostomy should be performed at an early stage. Special attention should be directed to the circulatory state since the sympathetic nervous system may be involved and there may be circulatory failure.

Tetanus. In tetanus the onset is usually less abrupt but the patient may not come under observation until a serious state has been reached. Muscle spasm may make it difficult to intubate the patient and a general anaesthetic with tubocurarine is likely to be needed. The muscle relaxant may have to be continued while the patient remains on artificial respiration.

Porphyria. In acute porphyria respirator management provides the only means of controlling respiratory failure and it may need to be continued for weeks. Care is required over the administration of drugs, as some, such as barbiturates, oestrogens and sulphonamides, may aggravate the disease. Drug administration is often the explanation for an acute episode. The mortality is high.

Myasthenia Gravis. Respiratory failure in this disease may be provoked by over-treatment with drugs, which may cause a cholinergic crisis, or the failure may be due to the disease itself. It is hardly ever a presenting symptom and usually there will be a background history of diplopia and muscle weakness. If the patient has not been treated with pyridostigmine or a similar drug, this should be administered and may relieve the respiratory difficulty. If treatment has already been given, it must be decided whether or not it is adequate or whether there is a cholinergic crisis. This can be resolved by administration of edrophonium chloride (Tensilon) intravenously. The initial dose should be small (2 mg) and may improve muscle power in the undertreated patient. If it does so, a further 8 mg can be given to confirm that the effect is convincing. If 2 mg fails to produce any improvement, caution is needed before giving additional doses, and the patient will usually require intensive respiratory care. Rapid administration of 10 mg of edrophonium to a patient on the verge of cholinergic crisis may precipitate a serious situation. If cholinergic crisis is confirmed it can be expected that respiratory assistance will be needed for several days at least, and often a week or two. It is better to institute respiratory care and to withdraw the cholinergic drugs to maintain the physiological state. An attempt to revert to voluntary respiration within a few hours of a cholinergic crisis nearly always fails and it is probably better to make a firm decision to continue with the respirator for at least 48 hours. This may be done with an endotracheal tube, but if after 48–72 hours there is no response to Tensilon, a tracheostomy will be needed. The untreated patient is likely to be profoundly weak but this does not matter while respiration is artificially maintained provided the patient understands what is intended.

The introduction of corticosteroid therapy may be considered, such as prednisolone 100 mg daily. Initially, this may depress respiration but it should certainly be considered if respiratory failure is prolonged. Patients with myasthenia are extremely sensitive to curare and may be made worse by streptomycin and kanamycin. The onset of respiratory failure in cholinergic crisis may be precipitated by infection, which should be treated by giving the appropriate antibiotic.

Respiratory failure in this disease is not always accompanied by severe muscle weakness and the opposite may obtain in which muscle weakness is severe but respiration adequate.

Status Epilepticus. This condition still carries a significant mortality and it is a matter of urgency to terminate the attack. In many cases there is a satisfactory response to intravenous diazepam, or paraldehyde intramuscularly. If control cannot be obtained with drugs within an hour, the patient is placed in considerable hazard. There is a risk from hyperpyrexia consequent on muscular contraction, and this may lead to brain damage. This aspect can be controlled by using tubocurarine and assisted respiration. Such treatment does not influence the cerebral dysrhythmia, which may be a cause of death. Anticonvulsant therapy should therefore be maintained. Several days of muscle relaxation with controlled respiration may be needed and it is convenient to give the relaxant by intravenous infusion. The dose is reduced from time to time to observe if there is any muscle twitching and the EEG may also help to predict the stage when the treatment can be withdrawn. If control of attacks has been maintained for a few hours within respirator or relaxation, the patient is unlikely to relapse in the course of the next day or two. It is, however, important to maintain the anticonvulsant therapy at this stage. Early treatment is vital, for delay may lead to circulatory collapse, renal failure and other complications.

Head Injury. Respiratory care has a limited place in the management of head injury. It must also be borne in mind that chest or cervical injury may be associated. In a comatose patient the possibility of intracranial haematoma requiring surgical treatment will, of course, be paramount. Prolonged respiratory care is seldom indicated.

Other Conditions. Occasionally, in *polymyositis* the muscles of respiration may be involved. The patient may be maintained on a respirator until the response to corticosteroid or other therapy is satisfactory. In other muscle diseases respiratory care is seldom indicated. Patients with *familial periodic paralysis* do not develop respiratory failure despite profound muscle weakness. Patients with *muscular dystrophy* may have respiratory problems at a late stage of the disease, when it may be questioned whether it is justifiable to assist respiration artificially. It might be indicated where an acute infection had produced a sudden deterioration in the patient's condition at an early stage in the disease, but if muscle weakness is profound and irreversible it may not be in the best interest of the patient to prolong the situation with a respirator. In cases of *drug overdose* (particularly barbiturate poisoning) assisted respiration may be useful. Such a situation may also arise in an epileptic patient who has taken an overdose of anticonvulsant. In *coma*, respiratory care may occasionally be required, at least until a diagnosis has been made; it is seldom long-term management in this way will be indicated.

Chronic Respiratory Disease, Cardiac Disease, Chest Deformity. In these patients the underlying disease may combine with the neurological disorder to produce effects that would not have arisen in a patient who was previously healthy. This may worsen the prognosis and must also be considered in the management. The help of the appropriate specialist will be needed in planning the best course of action.

The patient with pulmonary emphysema or central alveolar hypoventilation may present in coma, which is relieved by a period of assisted respiration.

Long-term Respiratory Care. Long-term care with a respirator presents many problems. It is demanding for the patient, for the relatives, and for the resources. Proper selection of patients for acute respirator care will to some extent reduce the need for long-term care. There are some patients who remain wholly or partly dependent on the respirator. This is seen particularly in patients with poliomyelitis, but also in the other neurological diseases that have been discussed. A few of these patients will have to remain in a respiratory unit, with all facilities at hand. In less severe cases it may be possible to use a simpler form of respirator such as the cuirass. This allows pressure and suction to be applied alternately to the chest wall and supports, rather than replaces, natural respiration. Some patients are able to sleep with the help of such a device and to manage without it during the waking hours. It is hazardous in those with bulbar palsy. The cuirass respirator may be helpful in states where muscle reserve is diminished, but it is not very efficient.

General Management. The onset of respiratory failure is alarming for the patient, and the distress may be increased when it calls for rapid action and intubation which deprives him of the capacity for speech. Matters of communication therefore become particularly important. It is necessary to explain what is involved, and to provide some means for the patient to communicate, such as writing, indicating from written or printed material, or gesture. Environment is important and the special unit here has the advantage that with all facilities at hand and trained staff it is easier to preserve a tranquil atmosphere. Most patients who have appreciated the benefits of assisted respiration rapidly settle down. Some, however, find it very difficult to tolerate the constraints placed on them, and sedation may then help. The patient is naturally fearful of being left unattended, hence there should always be an alarm system he can use. Extra support is needed at the time when the respirator is withdrawn. Confidence has to be regained. When assisted respiration is no longer necessary the tracheostomy tube may be replaced by a non-cuffed tube that can be occluded externally to allow speech. As the wound heals, this tube is withdrawn and the wound is then occluded with a simple dressing. Difficulties arise when repeated tracheostomy is needed. If this is judged to be likely, it may be better to leave the tube in position.

NEUROLOGICAL COMPLICATIONS OF CARDIAC ARREST

Cardiac arrest may be due to cardiac infarction, other heart disease, metabolic disturbances such as hyperkalaemia, or follow cardiac surgery. The effect will depend on the availability of prompt resuscitative measures, including cardiac massage and assisted ventilation. Cardiac arrhythmia may be reversible but the outlook is less favourable when there is asystole.

The commonest neurological complications are confusional states and coma. There may be focal neurological signs as well. A characteristic syndrome is intention myoclonus of the limbs arising as a result of cerebral anoxia. Some patients continue in a persistent vegetative state.

The possibility that anaesthetic drugs may be a contributory factor should be borne in mind, particularly after cardiac surgery. Improvement may be marked in the early stages and assessment over a period of 48 hours is advised.

Patients who remain unresponsive and require assisted respiration are unlikely to improve. Of those in coma not due to drugs the majority die within a year. Half of the 20 per cent who survive this period have neurological deficit.

CEREBRAL DEATH

The development of techniques to assist respiration and support the circulation, together with other aspects of intensive care, has raised problems of defining the moment of death. It may be possible to maintain the respiration, circulation, and some other physiological functions for some time after cerebral death. It is therefore necessary to consider the clinical and electrical criteria for defining cerebral death.

The problem of defining cerebral death is likely to arise in the setting of intensive care where the patient is supported by mechanical devices. An error is most likely to be made when the patient has taken an overdose of drugs or is hypothermic, remarkable late recoveries having taken place in this group. It is wise to make two examinations of the patient at an interval of not less than twelve hours.

Drug overdose and hypothermia must first be excluded. If brain death has taken place, there is no spontaneous respiration or movement over a period of three minutes. The pupils are dilated and do not react to light. Corneal, ciliospinal, gag, and brain stem reflexes are absent. There is no response to supraorbital pressure. The eyes move with the head; there is no doll's head movement. The eyes do not deviate in response to ice-cold water poured into the ear. Tendon jerks may still be present.

If the electroencephalograph is recorded, the tracing is flat, and the gain should be turned up to give an amplitude of 50 μV/cm. It is not necessary to have this information if the clinical features of brain death are present.

Difficulty arises in a few special situations, and it is possible for a patient with severe cortical deficit and an intact brain stem to continue for some weeks with spontaneous respiration and adequate circulation.

Turning off the Respirator. When the criteria of cerebral death have been satisfied the question of when to turn off the respirator needs to be answered. The reality of the situation may already be apparent, but a sympathetic discussion with the relatives is essential. If the matter is handled tactfully there is usually no difficulty in reaching agreement to turn off the respirator.

If the complete criteria for brain death are not fulfilled it may be necessary to wait for a longer period before the situation is clarified and it is accepted that there will be no recovery.

2

Rehabilitation

The object of rehabilitation, whether in relation to a head injury, stroke, or other neurological disorder, is to achieve the maximum degree of independence in the home, at work, or at school. This embodies the ideal that the patient is part of normal society even if the circumstances are changed.

The practice of rehabilitation medicine is an integral part of patient management in neurology and requires a team approach to achieve the best results. The basic team consists of the patient and relatives, nurse, doctor, physiotherapist, occupational therapist, speech therapist, and social worker. Many failures in rehabilitation are due to lack of communication between different disciplines. Unfortunately, the overall management is frequently at fault. In this chapter, the various disciplines a doctor must be familiar with if he is to achieve maximum benefit for his patient are introduced.

PHYSIOTHERAPY

The aim of physiotherapy is to obtain relief from pain and to assist in restoring muscle function. Various physical methods may be used to relieve pain, and muscle function may be improved by muscle strengthening exercises and exercises to improve the range of motion of the limbs and their co-ordination.

PHYSICAL METHODS

Heat. This is a well-tried method of relieving pain. Heat is applied by an infra-red lamp, diathermy, ultrasound, or by conductive methods such as water or wax baths. Heat is generally relaxing, it eases pain and assists in improving mobility.

The type of heat used depends on the individual problem but if a deep heat is required short-wave diathermy or ultrasound may be used. The kind of heat used and its indications are empirical. Cervical pain may be treated by simple heat from a lamp or infra-red heat. Pain from a frozen shoulder may be treated with short-wave diathermy. If heat is helpful it should be applied once or twice daily. Exposure should not be for more than thirty minutes, and around twenty minutes with short-wave diathermy. When heat reaches a certain intensity, it may be deleterious and cause local swelling and reddening of the skin.

Cold. The value of cold in neurological problems is restricted. The use of ice packs to spastic limbs produces a temporary increase in mobility but there is no convincing evidence that it is of any permanent value.

Massage. Massage has no real place in neurological practice, but may cause muscle relaxation in painful areas, and thus be of some value in pain relief.

Traction. Traction is more in the sphere of orthopaedic medicine than neurology. It is seldom applied in the presence of objective cord signs. Traction on the cervical or lumbar spine may be applied to relieve pain in the neck or back. It may be continuous or intermittent. If it is to work, the benefit will be felt early. Traction may be manual on the neck and, in some instances, this is sufficient to give relief. However, mechanical traction up to 55 kg on the neck, and up to 170 kg applied to the pelvis for low back pain, may be used.

Manipulation. Although it undoubtedly has a place in some acute spinal problems, the danger lies in indiscriminate manipulation without a definite diagnosis. Manipulation is the use of the hands in a suddenly applied force in the hope of improving joint mobility. Its main use is in acute lumbar spine problems. It should never be performed in the presence of objective neurological signs, and manipulation of the neck is likely to be dangerous when there is organic disease of the cervical cord.

Electrical Stimulation. This has been widely used in peripheral nerve injuries such as Bell's palsy. The idea is that daily electrical stimulation of denervated muscles prevents atrophy. If there has been complete denervation, there is no evidence that this is so, and if denervation is incomplete, the pattern of recovery will not be affected by electrical stimulation. Galvanic stimulation stimulates muscle and Faradic stimulation stimulates the peripheral nerve.

Hydrotherapy. This has value in increasing mobility in paralysed patients. Hydrotherapy eliminates gravity and increases mobility. Water can also be used to apply heat locally.

Exercises. Passive stretching exercises and exercises to improve muscle strength and mobility are an integral part of physiotherapy for neurological disease. There is a tendency to use physiotherapy as a psychological prop in chronic neurological disorders. Although physiotherapy may be of great value, complete recovery or a plateau must be achieved. When these stages are reached the course should end. It is important to recognise the indications for physiotherapy, otherwise the department becomes overloaded.

PHYSIOTHERAPY IN ACUTE NEUROLOGICAL LESIONS

In severe stroke, acute spinal cord damage or in a complete peripheral nerve lesion, the affected parts are immobile. The limb must be placed in an appropriate position to prevent contractures. When the lower limbs are affected, as in paraplegia or hemiplegia, the bed clothes must rest over a cradle. Footboards may be used to keep the foot at 90 degrees with the ankle, and some cushioning for the heel must be provided. The patient should lie relatively flat, with one pillow and foam rubber between the knees. Turning is required every two hours. Passive movements of the limbs are carried out throughout the joint range at least twice daily. This may be done by the physiotherapist or nurse. Cock-up wrist splints should be used selectively to keep the fingers and wrists extended.

As tone returns in upper motor neurone lesions the spastic limb must be regularly stretched throughout the range of movements. If spastic limbs are left unattended the limb adopts a contracted posture which, with the additional formation of fibrous tissue, makes free movement impossible.

In a hemiplegia the upper limb is in danger of contracting into an adducted, internally rotated position with the elbow flexed and flexion contractures at the wrist and fingers. In the lower limb, there may be contracture in an equinovarus position of the foot, flexion contracture of the knee and hip, and external rotation of the hip. Such postures must be avoided.

If little or no voluntary power returns to the paralysed limb the eventual posture is less important. However, it is obviously valuable to have the hemiplegic leg as straight as possible and to counteract severe foot drop with a below-knee caliper that has a toe-raising spring. A paralysed arm is best placed in a shoulder wrist sling. Sometimes full-length leg braces are used to assist in making a paraplegic patient more ambulant.

As voluntary power returns, great concentration is required to initiate minor movements. This is exhausting, and physiotherapy is best carried out in short repeated courses. The co-operation of the patient with the physiotherapist is important.

CHRONIC LESIONS

Upper Motor Neurone Disorders. In the established chronic neurological lesion, the emphasis must be on increasing voluntary control over movement, increasing sustained muscle strength, and improving co-ordination. Aids such as a below-knee caliper with toe spring, or walking frames or a tripod stick may be required.

In upper motor neurone problems with spasticity, willed movements return ideally against a background of full passive movement without permanent contracture. Thus, in the hand, the fingers will be capable of extending and the wrist extending despite the presence of spasticity. The situation may not be ideal and the correlation between spasticity and the ability to move is poor. At this stage the presence or absence of sensory disturbance and defects of co-ordination, as in cerebellar disease, have an important outcome on the eventual degree of independence.

Lower Motor Neurone Disorders. In muscle, root, or nerve disorders the object is to build up the power and endurance of the individual affected muscles by repeated exercise. Isometric or isotonic exercises may be used, but isotonic exercises provide more interest and variability for the patient.

In the example of a severe quadriceps weakness the programme may start with repeated knee-extension exercises without resistance. As strength is built up, weights are used to promote greater strength and maximum recovery. A pulley system can be used or weights or sand bags can be strapped to the foot. Although the affected muscle may remain partly denervated, maximum strength of the available muscle can be obtained. Where there is severe foot drop a below-knee caliper with a toe spring is helpful. Light, moulded, plastic splints worn inside the socks and shoes are in favour because of their cosmetic advantages but we find them relatively ineffective in severe foot drop.

OCCUPATIONAL THERAPY

The physiotherapist and occupational therapist work closely together. The public image of the occupational therapist as a person who helps to pass the patient's time in basket weaving misses the point of the speciality. Craft therapy is a facility used to reach a specific end.

The task of the occupational therapist is to work on the spontaneous or assisted improvement in muscle power and movement and to improve co-ordination and balance in a variety of ways. The ultimate object is to assess the patient's ability to live an independent daily existence at home or at work, and to advise and provide appropriate aids to assist in this aim. The occupational therapist is able to direct the patient into pastimes that will increase endurance such as standing and in improving arm hand co-ordination, and at the same time she will have to make some assessment as to the patient's mental abilities with regard to independence.

Assessment is therefore made at many levels. In daily living activities apart from the mental state, abilities to move within the home are looked at. The daily tasks of dressing, washing, bathing and feeding must be assessed. Cooking, laundry, shopping and the ability to cope with general family duties and outdoor activities are considered.

When problems are identified, attempts must then be made to rectify them. In some instances work under supervision in the department may increase independence. On the other hand, permanent disability has to be accepted. Various relatively simple gadgets may help to improve the situation.

Feeding aids include a Nelson knife or a suction egg cup. In dressing, elastic shoe laces may help. Bathing is made easier by a hand rail, a bath seat and board, and an elevated lavatory seat. The general layout of the house is important. A bungalow is ideal. If this is not possible, an extra stair rail, a chair lift, sliding doors and ramps are valuable.

It is important that the occupational therapist should be involved in the assessment and supply of special means of transport that will increase mobility. For those who are mobile but not able to use public transport, the combination of an invalid vehicle and self-propelling folding wheelchair is a great advance. For those who do not wish to have an invalid vehicle, a folding wheelchair for indoor and outdoor use is still a help. If the house is suitable, a battery-driven electric wheelchair can be applied for. At the present time, the patient must be unable to use a self-propelled chair to be eligible for an electrically propelled chair in the United Kingdom.

A mobility allowance has recently been introduced. It is available to those who are unable to use public transport. The invalid vehicle is being phased out. Those who have an invalid car are not entitled to a mobility allowance. At the present time the future of transport facilities for the disabled in the United Kingdom is in a state of flux. The current situation is summarised in Appendix 2. Regulations vary in Europe and the United States.

In the UK applicants for driving licences are required to declare whether they suffer from a certain disability. This includes epilepsy, severe mental subnormality, disabling giddiness or fainting, defective eyesight (inability to read a registration mark on a motor vehicle at 75 ft (22·9 m) with letters and figures 3½ inches (89 mm) high).

If these conditions are likely to cause danger on the road and are present at the time of application they are termed relevant disabilities. A prospective disability is a disorder such as muscular dystrophy or multiple sclerosis which may become a relevant disability because of the progressive nature of the disease. Prospective disabilities should also be declared.

In the case of a prospective disability the licence holder may be granted a licence only for a limited time and his fitness to drive may be reviewed by passing information from his doctor to the Medical Advisor to the Licencing Centre.

In general, a patient with a mild neurological disturbance has no difficulty in driving, but if any doubt exists, then an examination should be made with the patient in a vehicle. Adaptation to hand controls may make it possible for driving to continue. Each individual neurological condition requires separate consideration, and no firm rules can be laid down.

Many of the housing modifications and aids referred to above may be provided by the Social Services Department of local authorities and there must be a close link between the occupational therapist and social workers. The social worker is in a position to assess the progress and independence of the patient after discharge. In an ideal situation there should be a community nurse attached to each neurology unit, and a social worker. They can then liaise with their hospital colleagues and ensure continuity of care at home. Many people need to be advised about the availability of an attendance allowance for relatives or others who devote their time to looking after severely disabled people.

SPEECH THERAPY

Speech therapists have the task of assisting the disabled patient to interpret his external environment whether it be verbal, written, or from some other sense, and to express himself in verbal, written communication or by gesture, in a meaningful way. The speech therapist is therefore involved in much more than speech. There needs to be an understanding of the total neurological disability and whether it is progressive or static. If one merely confined oneself to an assessment of the number of speech therapists required to treat dysphasic stroke patients, this would outnumber those available for the treatment of all speech problems in the United Kingdom. A cynical viewpoint is that the speech therapist does no better with the patient than an intelligent well-motivated amateur, ideally a member of the family. There is little hard evidence to support the value of the speech therapist versus the amateur once assessment has taken place, but there is no doubt that the skills required to pin-point the various defects of higher cerebral function requires trained therapists, who may then pass on advice to relatives and friends.

SPEECH THERAPY IN CHILDHOOD

This is not really a matter of rehabilitation but of establishing speech that has been delayed in development for various reasons. The field is a wide one and includes the mentally subnormal child, the severely or partially deaf child, social deprivation, developmental dysphasia (central deafness), dyslalia and various types of dysarthria which may be accompanied by evidence of organic brain disease. Stammering is another important symptom requiring therapy.

It would be inappropriate to discuss all these subjects in detail. The problems involved differ widely. One of the most important points is to decide the reason for delayed speech, which may be multifactorial. Severe deafness may be diagnosed early by lack of response to simple manoeuvres in a baby clinic. High-tone deafness and partial deafness affecting high and low tones may be detected by audiometry. In all cases of deafness defects in articulation are prone to occur and severe sensory deprivation will impair the development of internal thought and language functions. Binaural hearing aids should be used in all deaf children.

The progress made in severe mental retardation depends on the ability of the child to imitate sounds and associate meaning with them. Severely retarded children do not normally develop meaningful speech.

Social deprivation often associated with some degree of subnormality may result in marked improvement in speech when the child is brought into a play group at a language school and stimulated.

Defects of articulation improve spontaneously as with dyslalia and regular treatment is not normally needed. In developmental dyspraxic speech disorders, only careful repetitive and imitative exercises will produce results. Improvement may be slow. Children with spastic dysarthria due to cerebral palsy respond poorly.

The concept of central deafness, which can be equated with developmental receptive and expressive dysphasia, presents serious problems. In these children, cortical evoked potentials may be elicited thus eliminating the possibility of disease in more peripheral pathways. The child may hear sounds but fail to appreciate them, with a subsequent disturbance of internal language and speech. Other children appear to comprehend but cannot speak normally. Developmental sensory dysphasia is a very difficult problem to manage. The otherwise normal intelligence of the child will distinguish it from mental subnormality. Continuous emphasis on sound recognition and differentiation is the basis of treatment. In the case of expressive defects language must be built up gradually by patient repetition of words, phrases, and sentences.

Stammering is a vast and controversial subject. The types are various. Basically there is a defect of the rhythm of voice production with abnormal breathing patterns. Treatment is a slow process, but there may be spontaneous improvement. The child should be instructed in regular, spaced, precise speech that is unhurried. Attending elocution classes may be helpful.

DYSPHASIA

Assessment. Dysphasia is a disability of widely varying severity and with a number of causes. The speech therapist is mainly concerned with dysphasia following strokes, head injury and benign or relatively benign tumours. The disability may vary from an ability to find the appropriate word on occasions to severe dysphasia with receptive and expressive components.

The object of assessment is to obtain a picture of the patient's abilities in the cognitive and expressive fields. The ability to read words and letters and name them, or to read them but not be able to name them are tested. Responses to varieties of verbal communication from simple commands to complex ones are tested. Cerebral dominance and the ability to write with the paralysed or non-paralysed hand are noted. A total picture of the disability is built up. One popular test is the Schuell test. This evaluates language function in the verbal and visual fields and by a series of tests isolates the problems in the individual. The patient may be found to have difficulties in verbal and visual recognition. Spontaneous speech may be greatly reduced but comprehension relatively well preserved. Speech may be fluent but gibberish with severe lack of verbal comprehension. The object of speech therapy is re-education of language function using the least damaged aspects of cerebral function.

Therapy. Long-term improvement in dysphasia may continue for two years or more. The results are better in the young and the left-handed. The latter is because of a tendency for left-handed people to have incomplete cerebral dominance for speech. Patients with severe disturbance of comprehension do not, in general, do well.

After assessment, a series of consultations takes place between the therapist and the patient. If comprehension is reasonable, but there is a severe disorder of motor expression, the therapist concentrates on re-educating motor speech. This is done by repeated pronunciation of words by the therapist and imitated by the patient. It may be helpful for the patient to feel the therapist's lip and tongue movements. Gradually a word vocabulary is built up and sentence construction attempted. Fatigue is common and sessions should not be prolonged.

When the patient has difficulty in naming objects, clues may be supplied by various pathways. A picture of an orange can be presented alongside the word orange printed on a card. An orange may be placed in the hand to provide a tactile clue. The ability to identify objects is built up using picture and word cards. Subtle differences can be used to try to build up a sentence structure, such as showing pictures with 'dog lying down' and 'dog standing up'. Pictures with multiple objects on them are used, as also can a series of cards with the names of each object on them so that the patient points to the picture relevant to the word and names it.

When there is considerable impairment of understanding the therapist has to attempt to teach the patient to understand simple words both spoken and written. The hope is that with gradual increase in word understanding more appropriate speech will result.

Group therapy is of value when a certain stage of competence is reached. The use of a mirror is valuable in patients with expressive disorders.

DYSARTHRIA

Dysarthria is a disorder of articulation and may result from a wide variety of diseases. From the point of view of speech therapy the field is limited. It is unusual for patients with extra-pyramidal disease to benefit from speech therapy and the drugs now available have assisted associated speech disorders.

The treatment of the dysarthria due to cerebellar disease is disappointing. Although repetitive exercises in word and sentence pronunciation can be given, the end results are disappointing. Multiple sclerosis is a common cause of this type of dysarthria and the condition is frequently progressive.

Spastic dysarthria may occur following head injury or cerebrovascular disease. The prognosis for speech improvement is better after head injury. Such patients may have a mixture of dysphasia and spastic dysarthria. The basis of therapy is the retraining by repetition of word pronunciation using a mirror and observing the therapist's lip movements. Slowly sentence structure can be built up. Although spastic speech is likely to remain after a severe head injury, adequate communication is usually possible.

NEUROLOGICAL NURSING

Among the staff of a neurological unit, none is more important than the nurse in the rehabilitation of a patient. The variety of disorders dealt with vary but she must be observant, methodical and with a sense of humour to survive the vagaries of the patient with a disturbed mental state.

The nurse is in contact with the patient for longer periods than anyone else, and she has much useful observation material to contribute. This may vary from the description of a seizure to the fluctuations in gait of the hysteric and the behaviour pattern of someone with presenile dementia.

Much of the rehabilitation work is done by the nurse. Passive physiotherapy, walking the patient down the ward, supervising the first proper bath and giving general encouragement all fall into the normal day's work. The nurse is the person who turns the patient every two hours and who prevents pressure sores. The standard of neurological rehabilitation always falls when nursing numbers and skill are inadequate.

In any neurological unit there must be regular discussion periods between the nursing and medical staff outside normal ward rounds and once a week there should be a time for discussion of relevant patients between the medical and nursing staff, the physiotherapists and occupational therapists and, preferably, a social worker and community nurse attached to the unit.

3

Psychiatric Aspects of Neurology

Psychiatry and neurology are closely related. The distinction between the two specialties is artificial, diseases such as depression and schizophrenia probably having an organic basis although the term functional psychosis is often applied to them.

Approximately 15 per cent of patients first attending a neurological out-patients department have a primary psychiatric problem, the actual proportion depending on selection. Such patients complain of somatic symptoms but have no organic disease. They may be depressed, anxious, or suffering from a personality disorder. In addition to this group of patients many chronic organic neurological problems are associated with a depressive illness, which may require treatment with antidepressant drugs.

Another problem is the presence of a functional overlay in patients with organic disease. This produces a greater degree of disability than would be expected on the basis of the organic picture. Thus, patients with the same disease may vary widely in their disabilities despite the similarity of their physical signs.

Patients with organic psychoses may be referred initially to a psychiatric unit emphasising the need for awareness of the presence of physical disease in patients with psychiatric symptoms.

MANIA

The term bipolar affective psychosis refers to patients who swing from mania to depression. Unipolar affective psychosis involves predominant depression or mania, but pure mania is rare. Unipolar endogenous depression is the commonest of the affective psychoses and in some patients features of depression and mania may coexist.

Clinical Features. In mild hypomania the patient feels well and is full of joy and exciting ideas and plans. There is considerable physical overactivity and mental thought flows at an alarming rate. The patient often becomes irritable if his plans are thwarted. Eventually, activity may become disorganised and purposeless, speech breaks down into rapid disjointed words and sentences and 'flights of ideas' appear. Severe insomnia occurs. In the most severe cases delusions, mental confusion, and clouding of consciousness supervene. The manic psychosis must be distinguished from the acute onset of a schizophrenic illness and an organic psychosis resulting from a brain tumour, encephalitis, or drug intoxication.

Treatment. Severe mania requires hospital admission. A phenothiazine such as chlorpromazine 50 to 100 mg intramuscularly given six-hourly may be used, but haloperidol is more effective. A dose of 5 mg intravenously may be given six-hourly until the patient is much quieter, and oral maintenance in a dose of 1 to 2 mg eight-hourly. Larger doses may be required.

For patients who frequently relapse, lithium carbonate may be used. Details of this drug are discussed below.

A short course of electro-convulsive therapy (ECT) is occasionally necessary but should be reserved for refractory cases.

Lithium Carbonate. This is used as a mood stabiliser and for treating patients with depression who have frequent relapses and those who swing from depression to mania. Although valuable it is a toxic drug. In acute mania 1600 to 1800 mg daily gives a serum level of 0·9 to 1·4 mmol/litre. A level of 1·5 mmol/litre is the maximum desirable. The blood lithium must be checked regularly. The toxic effects include muscle weakness, ataxia, and excessive thirst and polyuria. At levels above 1·9 mmol/litre consciousness is impaired.

DEPRESSION

There is no universally agreed classification of depression. The distinction between endogenous and reactive depression is not always possible. Patients with obvious environmental problems may still have a depressive illness and this may be an endogenous depression masked by other factors. Bereavement is an example of reactive depression.

Clinical Features. In a neurological context somatic symptoms due to depression are common. Headache, dizziness, neckache, backache, and generalised feelings of weakness occur. There may be no overt complaint of depression but lethargy, motor retardation, sleep disturbance and irritability if present make the diagnosis easier. If headache is a complaint it is frequent and severe and may not respond to simple analgesics. Tension headache may be associated with pain described as a tight band in the frontal and occipital regions or a pressure feeling over the vertex.

Differential Diagnosis. An endogenous depressive illness must be differentiated from an anxiety state and from a reactive depression that is clearly related to environmental problems. Organic neurological disease may be mistaken for depression and a cerebral tumour can be missed if consideration has not been given to organic possibilities. It may be difficult to separate depression from early dementia, as in both instances performance on psychometry may be abnormal. Clinically, the distinction can be difficult, but repeated examination of higher neurological functions by the clinician may eventually solve the problem. Sometimes early dementia comes to light when treatment for depression has been unsuccessful.

The reverse situation may come about when gross retardation and apparent intellectual failure are due to endogenous depression and not dementia. This is of particular importance in older age groups. It is difficult to lay down hard and fast rules for differentiating the two, clinical experience being the most important factor. The presence of a normal electroencephalogram is helpful, for in severe dementia the EEG is frequently abnormal. The distinction is of importance in view of the therapeutic implications.

Antidepressant Drugs. A number of effective drugs are available for treating depression. They fall into two main groups, the tricyclic antidepressants and the monoamine oxidase inhibitors. The neuropharmacology of depression is not fully understood but it is thought that one of the primary disorders in depression is depletion of central catecholamines. The monoamine oxidase inhibitors are thought to act by inhibiting the breakdown of noradrenaline in the terminal axon. Tricyclic antidepressants prevent reabsorption of noradrenaline from the synaptic cleft.

Monoamine Oxidase Inhibitors. These drugs were widely used for treating depression but since the dangerous side effects from paroxysmal hypertension with severe headache have been recognised, they have fallen into disrepute. When they are taken, food substances containing tyramine, such as cheese, red wine and broad beans, have to be omitted from the diet. There is, also, drug interaction with substances such as ephedrine and pethidine. If these dangers are appreciated, monoamine oxidase inhibitors are useful in treating atypical forms of depression where somatic symptoms are prominent. Tranylcypromine 10 mg t.d.s. and phenelzine 15 mg t.d.s. are two monoamine oxidase inhibitors in use. Tranylcypromine is frequently combined with trifluoperazine because of its stimulant effect. Both drugs may cause insomnia.

Some clinicians combine tricyclic antidepressants with monoamine oxidase inhibitors in refractory problems. A gap of 10 to 14 days between usage of the two types of therapy is generally recommended. It is accepted that in occasional circumstances combination therapy may be justified but this is best left to units accustomed to monitoring such situations. It is not advised in ordinary neurological practice.

Tricyclic Antidepressants. These are widely prescribed and are frequently effective. Many products are on the market but there is little evidence that one is superior to another. It is best to adopt a few well-tried drugs and gain experience in their use. In general, this group of drugs may be divided into those with or without a sedative effect. In prescribing them it must be realised that dosage requirements may vary enormously and one of the commoner clinical errors is underdosage. These antidepressants produce anticholinergic side effects such as dry mouth, visual blurring, and constipation, and they tend also to produce tachycardia and impotence and postural hypotension. The side effects vary from drug to drug and with individual response.

Imipramine and desipramine are two well-tried drugs that have no sedative effect. They take 10 to 14 days to become clinically effective. The basic dose is 25 mg three times daily. However, the dose requirement may be as high as 400 mg daily, although many physicians would be reluctant to go over 200 mg daily. In the high-dose ranges there may be sweating, involuntary movements of the jaw, and tremor. If used in agitated patients these drugs need to be combined with an anxyolytic agent such as diazepam. Treatment needs to be continued over a long period otherwise the relapse rate is high. The cycle of a depressive illness may continue for two years or more. Sometimes sudden weight gain heralds the end of the current illness and, in general, patients put on weight while taking them.

Trimipramine has a considerable sedative effect and is useful in treating patients with a marked sleep disturbance. It is not ideal if the patient is grossly retarded. Its chief value is in a patient in an agitated depressive state with sleep disturbance. The dose regime is similar to that outlined above. It is common to give the whole daily dose at night and can apply to with all tricyclic antidepressants.

Clomipramine also has some sedative effect. It is claimed to be particularly effective if phobic symptoms predominate. An intravenous form is available that can be used if quick results are required in the severely depressed. The drug should be given in a solution of 500 ml dextrose saline over half an hour to avoid its irritant effect on veins. The patient should rest after the infusion as drowsiness and hypotension are common.

Amitryptyline is well tried and effective. It has some sedative effect, but may need combination therapy with diazepam. The dose regime is similar.

Electroconvulsive Therapy. ECT is widely used in psychiatric practice. Some concern has been expressed about the frequency with which it is given for depressive illness. Before the advent of effective antidepressants, ECT was invaluable and restored normal mental health in a remarkable manner. The modern drugs available have reduced the need for ECT and a more critical approach is required with regard to the indications for its use. It is of considerable value in the severely retarded depressed patient and in the suicidal. Now that convulsions are modified by anaesthetic and muscle relaxants, crush fractures of vertebrae are very rare. Nevertheless, repeated courses of ECT cause memory failure and eventual intellectual deterioration.

Depression Associated with Neurological Disorders. In chronic neurological disease depression is common. In many instances it is a reaction to a distressing physical situation. The patient's basic personality is reflected in reaction to disease, and in purely reactive depression sometimes combined with an inadequate personality, drug therapy is of little value. Endogenous depression is seen in chronic neurological disease such as multiple sclerosis, Parkinsonism, and chronic epilepsy. When in doubt about the possible existence of endogenous depression a trial with antidepressants is justified. Regular discussions covering physical, social and emotional problems are important. It is necessary to bear in mind that the relatives of the sick patient may become depressed and require treatment themselves.

PERSONALITY DISORDERS AND NEUROLOGICAL DISEASE

Any physical illness must be influenced by the patient's basic personality and, indeed, psychopathy can result in social habits that result in neurological problems, as in alcoholism. It is convenient to group a number of personality reactions under this heading apart from hysteria and psychopathy. Anxiety reactions and a simple inability to cope with life stresses are all part of the disease process influencing functional disability and neurological disease. The term functional overlay is used to imply an excessive disability in relation to a disease process that cannot reasonably be attributed to direct physical causes. Some neurological symptoms and disabilities are purely functional and not associated with a specific disorder such as depression. For reasons that often remain obscure, patients may continue to complain of chronic backache and neckache despite all attempts to rehabilitate them. Sometimes these pain syndromes follow trauma, and compensation may be involved.

Anxiety. Anxiety is a common symptom that may cause tension headache and complaints such as dizziness, light-headedness and vague sensory and motor complaints. A patient often becomes anxious about the cause of a symptom such as headache, and fear of brain tumour or a cerebral haemorrhage is common. Reassurance with the minimum of investigation is often effective.

An enormous number of people take some form of tranquilliser and many drugs are available but it is best to use a few well-tried forms of medication. Although barbiturates have been widely prescribed in the past they have no real place in the modern therapeutics of anxiety. Barbiturate addiction is a troublesome problem and for that reason the benzodiazepine group of tranquillisers should be preferred. The most widely used drugs in this group are diazepam, chlordiazepoxide, and medazepam. In equivalent dosage there is little basic difference between them. Diazepam has greater anticonvulsant and muscle-relaxant properties. Diazepam is used in a dose range of 6 to 30 mg or more a day to alleviate anxiety. Chlordiazepoxide from 15 to 60 mg, and medazepam up to 30 mg daily. There is a wide variation in tolerance, although the only troublesome side effect is drowsiness. Sometimes very large doses are required.

Phenothiazines may be used to treat anxiety but are better left for conditions where anxiety accompanies a psychotic illness. Chlorpromazine and trifluoperazine are two widely used drugs. The dose requirements vary. Chlorpromazine 50 mg six-hourly, or trifluoperazine 1·5 mg eight-hourly may be used. Much higher doses are usually required to control psychotic symptoms.

Haloperidol may be used in the treatment of anxiety. A dose regime of 0·5 to 1·5 mg twice daily is a usual starting dose. Haloperidol and the phenothiazines have extrapyramidal side effects and produce dyskinesias.

It is not always possible to alleviate anxiety with drugs. The natural anxiety of a young woman who knows she has early multiple sclerosis is normal and only when such symptoms seriously interfere with daily living should medication be prescribed.

Phobias. Fixed phobic symptoms can ruin everyday living. The symptom may be isolated and specific such as fear of water or flying. In severe phobic states the patient may demonstrate a level of heightened anxiety and be unable to leave the house or travel alone. A phobic symptom often appears against the background of an obsessional personality.

When assessing the patient with phobias the possibility of an underlying depressive illness should be considered. Some patients respond quite rapidly to large doses of tricyclic antidepressants; for others, psychotherapy and behaviour therapy should be tried in an attempt to overcome the more specific types of phobia.

Insomnia. This is a common symptom in patients with chronic organic illness as well as in those who are anxious or depressed. The anxious person has difficulty in going to sleep. In endogenous depression early morning waking is a feature. In depressive sleep pattern a tricyclic antidepressant with sedative properties may suffice. There is no place for barbiturates as hypnotics today, and methaqualone is addictive. The benzodiazepines and chloral hydrate are useful. Nitrazepam 5 to 10 mg at night is popular and often effective as a hypnotic. The chief disadvantage is a gradual reduction in hypnotic efficacy which is common to all benzodiazepines. Flurazepam up to 60 mg is similar to nitrazepam, and diazepam may also be used. Chloral hydrate is an excellent hypnotic at all ages, but its chief disadvantages are an unpleasant taste and a gastric irritant effect. A dose of 2 g at night is usually effective. Dichloralphenalzone 650 to 1300 mg is palatable and useful in the elderly.

Hypochondriasis. Hypochondriasis presents an intractable problem. Once reassured about one symptom the subject usually returns with another and medication is not often of value, provided that underlying depression has been excluded. Reassurance is all that can be given. Hypochondriasis should be given the minimum of medical attention.

Compensation Neurosis. The 'postconcussional' syndrome and compensation neurosis form a subject of major importance because of the considerable amount of time lost from work after minor head injuries.

The characteristic symptoms are headache, dizziness, nervousness and irritability and loss of concentration. The symptoms are prolonged and often explained on the basis of malingering and a conscious desire for profit. It is likely that some patients who complain of such post-traumatic symptoms have an underlying neurotic personality or have been under stress at the time of the accident, which has subsequently been exacerbated.

An additional element is that minor head injuries may produce disturbances of vestibular function which can be recorded objectively, and the brain disturbance underlying concussion may reasonably be expected to impair concentration for some time.

Some of the patients respond to benzodiazepine drugs and, occasionally, antidepressants. This supports the view that malingering is not a common cause of compensation neurosis. It is a complex subject that requires an individual approach, and doctor bias is liable to prejudice conclusions. Further mention of the subject is made on page 145.

Psychopathy. This term covers a wide variety of disorders of personality and where the definition begins and ends is a matter of opinion rather than hard fact. Inadequate psychopaths may produce anxiety and phobic symptoms in relation to normal life stress. Aggressive psychopaths have unstable temperaments and may have rage reactions and be violent. Abnormal sexual behaviour also occurs. Psychopathy is untreatable. Sometimes side effects following alcoholism or drug addiction require more specific treatment.

Hysteria. Since the days of Charcot the identity and nature of hysteria has caused much controversy. While some dispute the definitive identity of hysteria as an illness, few would doubt that there are classical conversion symptoms and signs which are frequently neurological. The diagnosis is a 'dangerous' one to make, particularly in the older age groups. Many organic diseases such as brain tumour and subdural haematoma have been given the wrong label. In younger people multiple sclerosis and myasthenia gravis may be misdiagnosed as hysteria because of vague symptoms.

In making a diagnosis of conversion hysteria, one implies that the symptoms and signs are not consciously simulated as opposed to malingering. Blindness, deafness, dysphonia, paraplegia with or without bizarre sensory signs are some of the neurological features. Careful clinical examination should distinguish organic from hysterical disease although the picture may be a mixture of the two.

In hysterical blindness, the pupils will be of normal size and react to light. The visual fields are bizarre. In paraplegia, paralysis may be total but the reflexes present and normal. In incomplete paraplegia, muscles may contract in one situation and not in another. Disturbances of sensation are common in hysteria. All modalities may be lost and the cut-off point is often at the level of a joint or down the midline of the body from head to trunk, abdomen and the appropriate limbs. The patient may not feel the sharpest pin inserted into the skin and deny sensation of a tight grip on the arm. Vibration sense may be lost to the midline on the skull. Knowledge of normal anatomy will make it possible to distinguish these bizarre findings from organic disease. Hysterical fits are most usual in adolescent girls and young women. The attack may consist of jerking limbs with closed eyes and apparent unconsciousness, or a drop attack with no convulsions. The episodes usually take place in front of an audience and are frequently seen in the out-patient or EEG departments. Genuine and hysterical fits may coexist and cause problems in adopting a suitable anticonvulsant regime.

The importance in diagnosing hysteria is to avoid unnecessary and harmful investigation and to reduce medical attention to the minimum. In children and adolescents the problem may be temporary and resolve with simple measures such as physiotherapy. In this group the symptoms may represent a mechanism of escape from a stressful situation. In adult life the outlook is much worse, and an invalid existence may be adopted with equanimity. If this happens the problem is incurable.

Schizophrenia and Organic Psychosis. Schizophrenia in the form of a functional psychosis seldom presents in a neurological department. However, one may be faced with the problem of distinguishing it from an organic psychosis in a general medical or neurological department or a psychiatric unit.

Temporal lobe epilepsy may be associated with periodic aggression, a fluctuating psychosis similar to schizophrenia or a chronic schizophrenic psychosis which shows no spontaneous variation. Successful temporal lobectomy for severe seizure problems may be associated with improvement in aggressive tendencies, provided there is a reduction in fit frequency. There may also be improvement in fluctuating psychosis. There is no evidence of improvement in the chronic schizophrenic patient with temporal lobe epilepsy. In this instance the operation should only be performed for seizures that fail to respond to prolonged courses of adequate treatment.

Organic psychosis may develop for various reasons. Metabolic causes such as hypoglycaemia, hepatic encephalopathy, uraemia and porphyria must be excluded. Disseminated lupus erythematosus and sarcoidosis may be associated with a psychosis. The presence of epilepsy, clouding of consciousness, and additional general or neurological signs help to distinguish organic from functional psychosis. The treatment of organic psychosis depends on the underlying disorder.

Phenothiazine drugs have made a major impact in treating schizophrenia. Chlorpromazine is widely used and although longer acting phenothiazines have been produced there is no evidence that they are more effective. 1000 to 1500 mg of chlorpromazine a day may be needed in schizophrenia and in this case a drug such as benzhexol, 4 mg three times daily, may be used to counteract extrapyramidal side effects. If jaundice results with chlorpromazine another phenothiazine such as trifluoperazine can be used. Depot injections of fluphenazine decanoate (Modecate) 25 mg intramuscularly every two to four weeks are commonly used in chronic schizophrenia. This may induce depression.

Electroconvulsive therapy is used in treating schizophrenia. Unfortunately ECT has deleterious effects on memory. This empirical form of therapy should be reserved for patients not responding to drugs, which applies to depression and schizophrenia.

Iatrogenic Psychiatric Problems. A wide variety of drugs in use in neurological practice may alter a patient's mental state. Phenobarbitone and mysoline may cause depression, and sulthiame is an anticonvulsant that may produce a psychotic state. Phenytoin on a long-term basis may produce mental change which can be reversed by the administration of folic acid, although the nature and extent of this is controversial. Drugs used for treating hypertension such as reserpine, methyldopa and clonidine may cause significant depression. This severely limits the value of reserpine.

Corticosteroids may cause psychotic illness in certain individuals whether the source is ACTH or oral preparations. Preparations containing levodopa may precipitate mania or depression in predisposed individuals and the administration of levodopa to patients with dementia may cause increased confusion. Amantadine has a narrow dose range and causes hallucinations if given in excessive dosage.

These are some examples of drugs used in medical practice that cause psychiatric symptoms, and it is salutory to note that drugs used in psychiatry to treat one symptom may exacerbate another. An example of this is the production of depression with long-acting phenothiazine preparations used in schizophrenia.

4

The Neurogenic Bladder

The majority of neurogenic bladder problems are due to lesions of the spinal cord or cauda equina. Some are associated with brain disease or peripheral nerve involvement. Many patients with multiple sclerosis have bladder symptoms at some stage in the disease. The symptoms are distressing to the patient and may be aggravated by infection.

In any patient with retention of urine the question of spinal compression may be pertinent and may call for urgent surgical treatment. When the disturbance is chronic and not amenable to surgery, management is directed to the relief of symptoms, control of infection, and drainage of the bladder. Chronic infection leads to renal failure.

Symptoms and Signs. The commonest early symptom is precipitancy of micturition. Pain associated with micturition suggests infection. Difficulty in emptying the bladder may precede retention of urine. Increased frequency of micturition may be due to excessive fluid intake, metabolic disorder, renal failure, infection, neurogenic disease, or a contracted bladder.

Incontinence of urine indicates failure of sphincter control, which may occur when the bladder is distended. In women, this must be distinguished from stress incontinence which is usually provoked by coughing or straining.

Abdominal palpation is an unreliable guide to bladder size. When retention is suspected, drainage by catheter and measurement of the residual urine is necessary. In addition to the general neurological examination it is important to test sensation over the sacrum and perineum, assess the tone of the rectal sphincter by digital examination, and elicit the anocutaneous reflex.

Differential Diagnosis. Incontinence of urine in the child may be due to persistent enuresis and may recur later under psychological stress. Nocturnal incontinence may also raise the possibility of epilepsy. The mentally retarded may neglect regular emptying of the bladder and present with incontinence. Incontinence of urine may be simply a consequence of limited mobility, particularly when there is precipitancy of micturition as well.

The importance of urgent surgical measures to relieve spinal compression or root compression has already been emphasised. In young women with acute retention of urine and no other neurological signs, psychological factors should be considered.

ANATOMY AND PHYSIOLOGY

The main contractile mechanism of the bladder is the detrusor muscle. The detrusor fibres are very long and pass across the midline. The muscular arrangement of the bladder neck produces opening of the urethra and closure of the uretric orifices during normal micturition.

The nerve supply to the bladder is from the parasympathetic system at the second, third and fourth sacral levels. Sensory fibres run with the parasympathetic system and subserve pain sensation in the bladder and urethra. The role of the sympathetic nervous system is less important. It is probably responsible for closure of the bladder neck during ejaculation. Some bladder proprioceptive impulses run with sympathetic fibres to the lower dorsal cord. The external sphincter is supplied by the internal pudendal nerves (S 2, 3, 4) and has associated sensory fibres.

The bladder acts as a storage reservoir. During filling, an increasing volume of urine is accommodated at constant pressure. When the volume of urine reaches about 400 ml there is a rapid rise in pressure and an urge to pass urine. Micturition can be temporarily inhibited by voluntary control.

Cystometrogram. A clinical recording of bladder pressure produced by urine or artificial fluids is termed a cystometrogram. A pressure measuring system within the bladder and recording apparatus are required. The retrograde instillation of sterile distilled water at a constant rate and pressure is satisfactory. In the normal bladder there is a flat curve until about 400 ml of fluid is present. In upper motor neurone lesions and local bladder irritation the cystogram shows a rapid rise in pressure with less than 100 ml of fluid. Cystoscopy is therefore essential. The curve may be reversed towards normal with intramuscular emepronium bromide but oral therapy based on this may not be clinically effective. In an atonic bladder due to a lower motor neurone lesion or outflow obstruction the flat curve is prolonged and there may be an overflow incontinence. The residual urine volume after micturition should not be more than 10 per cent of the normal bladder capacity.

TYPES OF NEUROGENIC BLADDER

Bladder muscle has intrinsic tone unaffected by denervation. Atonic bladders result from prolonged over-distension. The type of bladder problem depends on the nature of the lesion and the extent and rate of evolution. The level of the lesion is important but may be difficult to assess when spinal shock is present. The presence of anal and bulbo-cavernosus reflexes indicates sparing of sacral segments and suggests that reflex bladder function may develop.

Cerebral Lesions. The higher control of bladder function is complex and does not depend on single centres. A centre in the superior frontal gyrus has an inhibitory influence and lesions in this area due to an aneurysm of the anterior communicating artery or a tumour may cause involuntary and sudden incontinence. There may be no general impairment of mental function. Incontinence also occurs with dementia. Unilateral hemisphere lesions do not usually cause incontinence as the co-ordinating functions for bladder control are bilaterally represented.

Unconscious patients become incontinent when coma is profound. When consciousness is less depressed, retention of urine may occur and produce restlessness. Catheterisation will relieve the situation.

In general, the underlying cause for the cerebral lesions determines the outlook for improved bladder function. In ruptured anterior communicating artery aneurysms, there may be spontaneous improvement, and appropriate surgery will prevent haemorrhage. However, the cerebral causes of bladder dysfunction are often progressive and not amenable to treatment; continuous bladder drainage may then be necessary.

Spinal Lesions. There are three basic types of spinal bladder disorder: (1) the sacral or lower motor neurone bladder lesion; (2) the upper motor neurone or spinal reflex bladder; (3) the deafferented bladder met with in tabes dorsalis and diabetic neuropathy. This differs from the sacral or cauda equina bladder in that sensation is lost due to involvement of the fibres travelling with the sympathetic nerves as well as the afferent nerves in the sacral arc. As the deafferented bladder fills there may be no attempts to empty by straining.

When a spinal lesion develops above the level of the conus there is a gradual loss of voluntary inhibition of micturition with reduced bladder sensation. Eventually, a spinal reflex bladder may develop but residual urine is usual. In a chronic conus or cauda equina lesion the bladder has to be emptied by repeated straining or manual compression but there is a considerable residual urine because the bladder sphincter does not open normally.

ACUTE RETENTION OF URINE

In an acute neurological lesion whether at sacral or suprasacral level, the response is urinary retention. In a high lesion this is due to spinal shock and in a sacral lesion due to involvement of the reflex arc. The basic early management of all acute lesions is similar. Bladder drainage will be required. In complete lesions there is no pain and overflow incontinence may be delayed because of early oliguria in trauma. Over-distension must be avoided as it leads to dilatation of the upper urinary tract. Infection usually results from catheterisation and may be perpetuated by local inflammation and urethral stricture due to poor technique.

Spinal cord compression should receive immediate surgical relief. In spinal trauma this is not usually required, such patients being transferred to a paraplegic centre.

Catheterisation. The type of bladder drainage adopted will depend on personal experience and the facilities available.

Intermittent drainage had a poor reputation because of infection. The advent of better catheters and more scrupulous technique has shown that this method is effective and with a relatively low infection rate (Guttmann). Catheterisation will be necessary three times a day. The advantage of the technique is that reflex bladder function can be easily assessed. The main disadvantage is that few departments would have the medical staff necessary to use such a technique effectively.

Continuous catheterisation is satisfactory. Failures are due to incorrect equipment and poor technique. A plastic catheter such as the Gibbon type may be used in males. In practice we prefer to use a balloon catheter. In favour of the Gibbon type of catheter is ease of manipulation and low incidence of irritant effects, but it is difficult to maintain in position and should be changed twice a week. The Foley catheter is more easily retained but the balloon may produce local trauma, including bladder calculus and urethral ulceration. The male urethra must be sterilised by injection of an antiseptic jelly which can be retained for five minutes, using a penile clamp.

In women a balloon catheter is adopted (Foley). It must be of inert material.

Suprapubic drainage is used in traumatic paraplegia in some centres. In the absence of anatomical abnormalities of the urethra it seems to have no particular advantages.

MANAGEMENT OF CHRONIC BLADDER PROBLEMS

The acute lesion may show marked spontaneous improvement, as in early multiple sclerosis. If recovery does not take place attention will have to be paid to continuing satisfactory drainage, the management of incontinence, and the prevention and treatment of urinary complications. In sacral lesions attempts should be made to encourage the patient to empty the bladder by repeated straining and manual compression. Reflex micturition may be delayed for a long time and never be adequate.

Bladder training is particularly important for women. As soon as the patient can sit she should make regular attempts to micturate, by straining in the case of sacral lesions, and by suprapubic tapping in supra-sacral lesions. The residual urine is reassessed by catheterisation each day.

Use of Drugs. These may help in promoting bladder drainage or controlling incontinence.

Cholinergic drugs improve bladder emptying. Carbachol is given in a dose of 0·25 to 0·5 mg by subcutaneous injection, or 0·2 to 0·8 mg orally three times a day. Distigmine is a long-acting anticholinergic drug and can be given in a dose of 5 mg orally daily. Assessment of residual urine by catheterisation is necessary if these drugs are to be used. They are helpful in the treatment of the atonic bladder provided there is no outflow obstruction. If patients with retention fail to respond to carbachol the bladder must be catheterised without delay. Bethanecol chloride 10 to 30 mg t.d.s. orally is an alternative.

Anticholinergic drugs reduce the excitability of the uninhibited neurogenic bladder. Atropine sulphate 0·6 mg three times daily may be combined with propantheline 15–30 mg t.d.s. Emepronium, an antimuscarinic drug, may be used in a dose of 50 mg t.d.s. up to 600 mg daily. Imipramine has been used for incontinence because of its anticholinergic effect. The dose is 25 mg t.d.s. or 50 mg at night.

Operative Procedures. Bladder neck resection has a limited place in patients whose detrusor activity is insufficient to open the urinary outlet. It is thus used in appropriate patients with conus and cauda equina lesions. It may also help in diabetes mellitus, tabes dorsalis, and after surgical destruction of the sacral nerve supply.

Occasionally, the operation may be considered when a suprasacral lesion has not been associated with recovery of useful detrusor function despite progress in other directions. The resection is transurethral and may be performed in women as well as men.

Division of the external sphincter in the reflex suprasacral bladder is done to relieve spasticity. In the lower motor neurone bladder it is occasionally performed to overcome smooth muscle contraction which is thought to be under sympathetic control. These patients may already have had a bladder neck resection. This operation produces stress incontinence in the female and is of more value in the male.

Drainage in Chronic Bladder Lesions. If micturition is not satisfactory appliances will still be required. Urinary incontinence may be a problem even if reflex micturition is established. The condom type of urinal is effective in males. The condom should be replaced daily and the two drainage tubes once a fortnight. In females incontinence pads are helpful.

Continuing catheter drainage will be required in many women, and males who do not get on with a condom system. The techniques for catheter use have been described already. In a woman, care must be taken to avoid ulceration of the anterior wall of the urethra. The drainage tube should be taped to the thigh or abdomen to avoid traction.

Occasionally, special operative drainage techniques are required. Urinary diversion may be indicated for severe incontinence. Implantation of the ureters into an ileal or colonic conduit is the procedure employed. The operation is most satisfactory in spina bifida in females.

Electrical Stimulation. This is not established as a routine procedure in neurogenic bladder. Electrical stimulation of the pelvic floor muscles has been used in stress incontinence. Direct bladder stimulation to enhance detrusor activity has given rise to pain due to local spread of electrical activity. Contraction of perineal muscles by current spread produces urethral obstruction. Stimulation of sacral nerves may cause penile erection as well as contraction of the external sphincter.

A future place for electrical stimulation may exist in the management of lesions of the sacral centres and in producing controlled evacuation in suprasacral lesions.

URINARY COMPLICATIONS

Infection is common in association with a neurogenic bladder but it can be reduced by careful attention to catheter technique and avoidance of stasis. Acute hydronephrosis and pyelonephritis result from a blocked catheter or retention. Chronic renal lesions result from stasis and ureteric reflex.

Chronic infection may persist in the presence of bladder stones or renal calculus; the former is more likely when balloon catheters are used. Table 4.1 lists the antibacterial drugs commonly used in treating bladder infections together with some notes on characteristics and usage.

In general, symptomatic urinary infections should be treated, but it is debatable whether chronic asymptomatic bacteruria requires therapy.

SOME SPECIFIC NEUROLOGICAL DISORDERS

Spina Bifida (*see also* Chapter 15). Bladder involvement may be present at birth, or delayed. The usual type of involvement is the lower motor neurone type with paralysis of the detrusor and pelvic floor muscles. A mixed picture also occurs in which the reflex activity of the bladder is excessive and the external sphincter paralysed. A pure reflex bladder may develop.

A large number of infants with severe neurological defects are now surviving, and bladder care forms a substantial problem in management. In infancy the paralysed bladder is emptied by frequent manual compression. In the case of reflex bladder, napkins may be used, and in some instances it will be possible to have some control over reflex micturition when the child is older. In boys a condom can be worn. In severe incontinence in girls urinary diversion to an ileal or colonic loop is necessary.

If the urine becomes infected, catheter drainage is often required and consideration must then be given to bladder-neck resection or division of the external sphincter. Urinary diversion is necessary if there is evidence of progressive dilatation of the ureter and calyces.

Multiple Sclerosis (*see* page 122). The type of bladder disturbance varies. Precipitancy and urgency are the commonest clinical complaints and they may be helped by propantheline or atropine. Acute retention of urine may be caused by a suprasacral cord lesion or a sacral one. Frequently there is spontaneous improvement but catheter drainage will be required for several

Table 4.1. Antibacterial Drugs—Pattern of Sensitivity and Resistance

	E. coli	*Proteus mirabilis*	*Proteus (other strains)*	*Strept. faecalis*	*Pseudomonas aeruginosa*	*Klebsiella aerogenes*	*Comment*
Amoxycillin	S	S	R	S	R	R	More potent than ampicillin
Ampicillin	S	S	R	S	R	R	Telampicillin gives higher blood levels
Co-trimoxazole	S	S	S	S/R	R	S	Synergistic effect of two drugs
Sulphonamides	S	S/R	R	S/R	R	R	Mainly domiciliary use
Tetracyclines	S	S/R	R	S/R	R	R	Infrequently used now
Nitrofurantoin	S	S/R	R	S	R	R	Avoid in renal failure—neurotoxic
Nalidixic Acid	S	S	S	R	R	S/R	
Carfecillin	S	S	S	S	S	R	Expensive. Oral drug of choice for *Pseudomonas aeruginosa*
Cephalexin	S	S	R	S/R	R	S	Expensive. Useful in penicillin sensitivity
Carbenecillin	S	S	S	S	S	R	Parenteral drug of choice for *Pseudomonas aeruginosa*
Cephaloridine	S	S	R	S	R	S	Parenteral only. Useful in penicillin sensitivity
Aminoglycosides	S	S	S	S	S	S	Only use in severe resistant infection
Polymyxins	S	S	S	S	S	S	Only use in severe resistant infection

weeks. Satisfactory function may return or bladder symptoms persist. In practice, patients with advanced multiple sclerosis do not often benefit from surgical treatment except for transurethral resection in men with reduced detrusor activity. Most women with severe bladder problems are better with continuous catheterisation. Men may need only condom drainage provided residual urine is not excessive.

Tabes Dorsalis. This is now a rare disorder. Bladder sensation is lost, and the damage is to the sympathetic and parasympathetic afferent fibres. Because of the neglect of abdominal straining the bladder enlarges and the upper tract dilates. The patient must be instructed in regular attempts at evacuation. Surgical resection of the bladder neck is often helpful. There is a similar problem in diabetic patients.

Herpes Zoster. This may involve the sacral sensory root ganglia and, occasionally, the motor cells as well. An eruption on one side of the bladder wall is usually accompanied by a rash on the buttock. Bladder sensation may be heightened and there can be haematuria. In severe cases there is loss or impaired bladder sensation and retention of urine which requires catheterisation for a short period. Recovery is usual. In rare cases where function is not restored it may be necessary to consider measures to improve drainage.

5

Chronic Pain

The management of chronic pain is not the specific province of the neurologist; it covers the whole of medicine. In this chapter, specific painful disorders such as migraine and trigeminal neuralgia are omitted, the subject discussed being the management of long-term chronic causes of pain, and pain in terminal illness.

ANATOMY AND PHYSIOLOGY OF PAIN

There is no agreement about the anatomy of pain. The concept of specific receptors for all modalities of sensation is probably incorrect, and more emphasis has now been placed on the temporal and spatial patterns of stimuli reaching the central nervous system from peripheral receptors. The gate theory of pain, introduced by Melzack and Wall, has attracted support and has practical implications. This theory assumes that sensory impulses travelling up large myelinated fibres are in competition with stimuli from small myelinated fibres. The 'gate' is open or closed according to the excitatory or inhibitory effects of these stimuli. This leads to the view that counter stimulation of large peripheral fibres or the dorsal columns in the spinal cord may relieve chronic pain. Pain is perceived at thalamic level, although the cerebral cortex probably plays a part in discriminatory and emotional aspects.

Pain is perceived differently by each individual. The pain threshold depends on the state of mind and personality of the patient; as a symptom, it has strong emotional associations. The pharmacological actions of analgesics remain uncertain and this restricts our understanding of pain mechanisms.

THE RELIEF OF PAIN

Pain may be a temporary experience that requires no specific measures other than simple analgesics. Continuous chronic pain profoundly influences the outlook and mental state of the individual. The pain is often due to advanced malignant disease, life expectancy may be short, and the patient's general condition poor: in these circumstances, unless a simple effective operation can be performed the use of analgesics is preferred. Most analgesics have unwanted effects, and considerable care must be taken to choose the correct drug for the individual and give a minimal but effective dose. The frequency of dosage is most important. Dr Cicely Saunders in her work on the treatment of pain in terminal illness has shown that doses should be given at intervals that produce continuous freedom from pain so that the patient does not have to ask for relief. The regime must therefore be flexible. The addition of a psychotropic drug may allow reduction of the dose of an analgesic.

There are many physical methods for treating chronic pain, ranging from nerve or root section and cordotomy to the use of sclerosing injections. These techniques are effective when correctly selected.

DRUG TREATMENT OF PAIN

The number of analgesics now available is bewildering. Some are of value in malignant disease and chronic nervous tissue damage. In general, potent narcotic analgesics should not be used unless the patient has advanced disease with very severe pain. Less potent drugs can usually be given with good effect. Most patients prefer to take medication orally and long-term parenteral administration is very inconvenient.

The dose of any narcotic used must not be increased to a level at which the patient is troubled unnecessarily by side effects which may prove very distressing and destroy any chance of well being. Dizziness, dryness of the mouth, severe constipation, respiratory depression and sleepiness are common with narcotics. If the patient can be rendered pain free, mental alertness is to be preferred.

Mild Analgesics. These drugs are helpful in a wide variety of musculoskeletal pains and headache—

Acetylsalicylic acid (aspirin) is available in many forms. It is an anti-inflammatory drug when given in excess of 3·6 g daily. In smaller doses it is an analgesic that has its limitations because of unwanted effects.

Gastric erosion is the most deleterious and makes it unsuitable for long-term use as a simple analgesic. In high doses it causes tinnitus, dizziness, and mental confusion. It is excreted in the urine in conjugated form. The dose is 300 mg to 1 g four-hourly, orally.

Paracetamol is an alternative to aspirin. The possible adverse effects on renal function make long-term therapy in large doses undesirable. The dose is 325 to 650 mg four-hourly, orally. In overdosage, paracetamol causes severe hepatic necrosis.

Codeine phosphate is an opium alkaloid with weak analgesic properties. The average adult dose is 30 to 60 mg four-hourly, by mouth. It causes constipation and is seldom effective in chronic pain. It is often combined with aspirin.

Dihydrocodeine is a semisynthetic opium alkaloid that is well absorbed when given by mouth. It is twice as potent as codeine phosphate. The dose is 30 to 60 mg every four to six hours, orally. It causes nausea and constipation. Some patients find the nausea particularly troublesome. An intramuscular injection of 50 to 100 mg is effective.

Dextropropoxyphene is a useful mild analgesic. It is often combined with other drugs in proprietary preparations. The dose is 65 mg four-hourly by mouth. It may, occasionally, cause drowsiness.

Pentazocine is now widely used as an effective analgesic with about half the potency of morphine. Addiction is not a serious problem. The dose is 25 to 200 mg orally four-hourly or 30 mg intramuscularly four-hourly.

Dipanone is a diphenylheptane derivative. It is slightly less potent than pentazocine. It is normally combined with cyclizine. The dose is 10 to 25 mg six-hourly by mouth, or 25 to 50 mg intramuscularly.

Drugs used mainly in rheumatic diseases may help neurological patients with skeletal or joint pain. Naproxen, ibuprofen and flufenamic acid have anti-inflammatory properties. They cause gastric irritation but are now widely used as an alternative to aspirin in mild joint disease. Indomethacin is much more potent but there is a high incidence of gastric intolerance, dizziness, and headache. The daily dose is 25 mg t.d.s. but higher doses, particularly at night, may help joint stiffness. A combination of indomethacin 100 mg at night plus diazepam 10 mg is helpful. Phenylbutazone is an effective anti-inflammatory drug but may lead to agranulocytosis and aplastic anaemia. Its use should be restricted to patients with refractory joint pain.

Major Narcotics. These drugs must be used with great caution in non-malignant disease. They are seldom justified in chronic pain syndromes where life expectancy is considerable. Individual preferences will dictate which drugs are used, but extensive experience in the use of a few drugs is better than a policy of constant variation.

Pethidine, a piperidine derivative, is disappointing as a major analgesic. It is much less potent than morphine and side effects are common. Sickness, dryness of mouth and constipation are prominent. It does not have a euphoriant effect. The dose is 75 to 200 mg four-hourly by mouth and up to 200 mg by intramuscular injection. We do not recommend it and its short duration of action is a major disadvantage.

Methadone hydrochloride is a diphenylheptone derivative. It is useful as an oral analgesic and is as potent as morphine. The dose is 5 to 50 mg six-hourly, orally.

Parenteral morphine and diamorphine are the drugs of choice in severe terminal pain. Morphine by mouth is not satisfactory. In a starting dose of 10 mg four- to six-hourly, intramuscularly, morphine is regarded by many as the most useful parenteral drug. Nausea and vomiting may require treatment with antiemetics. In the United Kingdom diamorphine is often preferred. It is two to three times more potent than morphine but has a short duration of action. The drug is better absorbed by mouth than morphine and does not make the patient drowsy although a sense of well being is apparent. The oral dose is 4 to 8 mg three- to four-hourly. The starting parenteral dose is 5 mg and may gradually need to be increased.

The Brompton 'Cocktail' is a popular oral mixture for terminal illness. Morphine or diamorphine is the basic narcotic. The formula varies but we recommend, diamorphine and cocaine elixir BPC containing diamorphine 5 mg, cocaine 5 mg, alcohol (90 per cent) 0·625 ml, syrup 1·25 ml, and chloroform water to 5 ml. The alcohol may be in the form of whisky or gin. The amount of diamorphine may be increased as required and chlorpromazine can be added.

Psychotropic Drugs. Major and minor tranquillisers and antidepressants have an important part to play in relieving chronic pain. Anxiety and depression are common features in many painful conditions. Endogenous depression may be precipitated by a chronic illness and make the response to analgesics unsatisfactory. The pain of phantom limb, postherpetic neuralgia and intercostal neuralgia may all be helped by the combination of a phenothiazine with a tricyclic antidepressant. These drugs alter the reaction to pain rather than pain perception. Pericyazine, fluphenazine, chlorpromazine or perphenazine may be used. The antidepressants that may be combined with these phenothiazines is a matter of personal choice. We use imipramine, desipramine, amitriptyline, clomipramine and trimipramine. The doses of these drugs have been discussed in Chapter 3.

OPERATIVE AND CHEMICAL INTERRUPTION OF PAIN PATHWAYS

A variety of neurosurgical procedures is available to relieve severe pain. These operations may be performed in malignant disease, arachnoiditis, painful back and chest problems, phantom limb pain, causalgia, and pain that may occur in the body following destructive lesions in the central nervous system and peripheral nerves. Apart from operative techniques, chemical lesions may be made with phenol and alcohol. Local anaesthetic injections may be used to relieve local pain before more permanent measures are taken. An ethyl chloride spray on the skin or the injection of ice-cold saline intrathecally have also been applied, particularly in postherpetic neuralgia.

Peripheral Nerve Section. The section of peripheral nerves is of limited value. In trigeminal neuralgia (page 57), the infraorbital and supra-orbital nerves may be sectioned for severe pain. Relief. From these procedures seldom lasts for more than a year. In occipital neuralgia, often associated with upper cervical spondylosis, section of the greater and lesser occipital nerves at the base of the occiput may be tried. In meralgia paraesthetica there is seldom any need to carry out an operative procedure (page 194).

Root Section (rhizotomy). Persistent severe local pain due to involvement of spinal nerve roots may be amenable to posterior root section. The pain may be felt in local malignant disease of the chest, after thoracotomy, over operation scars, and in lumbar disc disease. Rhizotomy of posterior nerve roots will have no effect on amputation stump pain nor will it help postherpetic neuralgia.

If a posterior rhizotomy is to be performed the precise roots involved must be delineated. Some operative failures result from incorrect localisation or section of too few roots. At least one root above and one below the affected level must be divided.

Peripheral Nerve and Root Injection. Chemical damage to nerve roots may be achieved by using ethyl alcohol or phenol in oil. Injection of alcohol into nerves will cause destruction of axons and myelin sheaths; it was widely used for injection of the trigeminal ganglion in trigeminal neuralgia but thermocoagulation is replacing it.

Phenol. Phenol in glycerin (5 per cent) has now replaced alcohol injection because it is more effective. If it is combined with Pantopaque the injection can be made under radiological control. The technique is described on page 121). One of the most important uses of intrathecal phenol is in the relief of painful flexor spasms. Relief of pain is due to destruction of pain fibres but histological studies have shown degeneration in fibres of all diameters.

Phenol is a viscous heavy fluid and the solution requires warming before injection through a lumbar puncture needle. The complications of chemical nerve damage are anaesthesia, hyperaesthesia, motor weakness, and sphincter damage. Response is unpredictable and the initial injection should be small.

When phenol is used to block a peripheral nerve the exact course of the nerve must be localised by electrical stimulation of the needle. Intrathecal block for severe pain should be performed at the spinal level where the nerve root *leaves* the spinal cord. This level is one segment, or sometimes two segments, higher than the spinal level in the cervical cord, two segments higher in the dorsal cord, and three segments higher in the lumbar cord. The spinal needle should be left in position while 0·1 ml of 5 per cent phenol is injected. The effect on pain can then be assessed. All analgesics should have been withdrawn for twelve hours prior to the procedure.

Examples of the use of phenol are in trapped ilio-hypogastric nerve in scar tissue following hernia operation, intractable intercostal neuralgia, and pain in the arm due to malignant disease in the lung apex and supraclavicular fossa.

Local Anaesthetics. Local anaesthetic injections may give relief in certain neuralgic conditions. Occipital neuralgia may be eased by injection of anaesthetic into nodules in the trapezius muscles, and the benefit may be long lasting. Divisions of the greater and lesser occipital nerves when the neuralgia is related to cervical spondylosis has already been referred to. Local anaesthetic may also be used in supraorbital neuralgia; 1 per cent lignocaine is injected into the nerve as it runs over the supraorbital ridge. If successful, a more permanent block may then be achieved with phenol. Many cases of supraorbital neuralgia are due to idiopathic trigeminal neuralgia, although post-traumatic cases are also known.

Lumbar epidural block with a local anaesthetic may be valuable in relieving intense muscle spasm and back pain; 20 to 30 ml of 0·5 per cent lignocaine are injected at the L2–3 interspace. The L3–4 space may also be used. Manipulation of the back may be combined with the injection. This technique may produce prolonged and permanent relief of symptoms and can be repeated. The greater success is with acute back lesions.

Chronic disc disease does not respond so well, but a similar injection of lignocaine combined with 50 to 100 mg of methylprednisolone may be tried.

Antero-lateral Cordotomy. This operation is designed to cut spino-thalamic fibres in patients with intractable pain. It is usually performed at one of two levels. For pain below the mid thorax, including the lower limbs, the operation is carried out at the third thoracic segment. For pain above this level the lesion has to be at C1–C2. In the thoracic operation a cut to 5 mm may be made and 8 mm in the cervical region. Operations are best performed under local anaesthetic so that the patient can comment on the result. After an initial section, sensory testing should be carried out and if there is incomplete analgesia but no motor weakness the lesion may be extended.

Cordotomy may be used for pain in the lower limb caused by abdominal malignancy, or pain in the upper limbs due to malignant disease such as carcinoma of the breast and lung. However, it may be impossible to raise analgesia to a sufficiently high level with a cervical cordotomy. This may be combined with a posterior rhizotomy, or phenol injections can be used as an alternative.

Respiratory failure after high cervical lesions is the most serious complication. It is most likely to come about after a bilateral operation and when lung function is already impaired. Respiratory failure may be temporary, and facilities should be available for ventilator care in the first week after operation. Occasionally, sudden death from respiratory failure occurs at night. Hypotension is usually temporary. Elevation of the foot of the bed and a recumbent posture for the first postoperative week are the basic precautions. There may be retention of urine; this is more likely after bilateral operations and is usually temporary. Severe weakness is rare. Bilateral section is more likely to produce motor symptoms. Unpleasant sensations are experienced in 5 to 10 per cent of patients.

Cordotomy will relieve pain in 50 to 70 per cent of patients. After an interval of months or years the level of analgesia may fall, and pain returns. A repeat cordotomy is not often successful.

Percutaneous Cordotomy. This recently developed technique avoids open operation. Radiographic control is essential. A lumbar puncture needle is inserted to lie anterolateral to the spinal cord between the first and second cervical laminae. Electrocoagulation or radionecrosis may be used. The depth of the lesion will be determined by the length of time the probe is left in place. The operation has a lower mortality than classical cordotomy and it can be performed on patients who are unfit for major surgery.

Commisural Myelotomy. An operation to relieve pain by dividing spinothalamic fibres as they cross in the anterior commisure has been performed but it does not have wide appeal. A vertical incision is made in the median plane of the spinal cord. The level of the operation will determine the sensory loss, which is bilateral and symmetrical. The chief value of this procedure may lie in the treatment of bilateral pain from pelvic malignancy. Stereotactic commisural myelotomy has been performed in the cervical region.

Brain-stem Operations. High cervical cordotomy may not relieve pain in the upper limbs, and because of the need to relieve pain in the head and neck a variety of procedures have been performed on the brain stem.

Medullary tractotomy involves division of the spinothalamic tract at some point in the medulla. It may cause ataxia and has a mortality of 20 per cent. The operation is seldom performed. Pontine tractotomy has similar limitations.

Mesencephalic tractotomy at a level between the inferior and superior colliculi has been shown to relieve pain in the head and neck as well as the trunk and limbs. It is associated with a high incidence of unpleasant dysaesthesiae.

All these operations are difficult to perform and have a high incidence of side effects. Stereotactic mesencephalic tractotomy has proved successful but it is not widely performed.

Thalamotomy. Various stereotactic thalamic lesions have been used in the treatment of chronic pain. Relief from pain may be temporary, the success of operation relating to the site and extent of the lesion. Since the termination of pain pathways within the thalamic nuclei is complex a consistent attitude to operative localisation has not yet developed. Lesions in the main sensory ventral posterolateral nucleus cause marked sensory loss but little pain relief. Much better results are obtained with lesions in the parafascicular, intralaminar, and median nuclei. There is little sensory loss but good pain relief. It is particularly interesting that lesions placed in the anterior nuclei and the dorsal-medial nuclei produce alteration in pain reaction but no analgesia.

Thalamotomy for thalamic pain or malignant disease is slowly growing in popularity but the results are still unpredictable. The operation is relatively safe and has a mortality of about 3 per cent.

Leucotomy. Leucotomy has not gained wide acceptance for pain relief. Cingulotomy, inferior medial quadrant frontal section, and unilateral leucotomy produce an alteration in affect and reaction to pain but there is the possibility that more striking changes take place in the mental state. Such procedures are difficult to justify.

MISCELLANEOUS PROCEDURES FOR PAIN RELIEF

CSF Barbotage. This is the withdrawal and replacement of cerebrospinal fluid for the relief of pain. Ice-cold saline was originally used to replace the cerebrospinal fluid, and temporary relief has been reported in postherpetic neuralgia. Reinjection of the patient's own cooled spinal fluid has also been tried but this technique does not have wide application. It may be applied in postherpetic neuralgia, when the injection should be made in the region of the pain. It may also be tried for malignant disease causing pain in the lumbar region. When ice-cold or hypertonic saline is used a general anaesthetic is required.

Sympathectomy. The operation of sympathectomy may be performed at various levels and is useful in the treatment of causalgia and severe pain due to visceral disease. In the latter, operation will be ineffective if malignant disease has spread beyond the capsule of the organ concerned. This limits its practical value. The use of sympathectomy in causalgia is discussed on page 196.

Electrical Stimulation. Recent developments involve electrical stimulation of large A fibres in peripheral nerve, thus blocking transmission through the smaller C fibres. The technique has been modified for stimulation of the dorsal columns of the spinal cord.

In nerve stimulation the electrodes are placed over the affected part. A battery-operated generator supplies the stimulus source. The current is turned up until a mild tingling is felt, the frequency and duration of the impulses then being adjusted to produce a suitable stimulus of a mild tingling type over the painful area. It has been used for amputation stump pain, neuromas, and postherpetic neuralgia. The electrodes can be implanted beneath the skin or directly over the posterior columns.

These techniques are not yet established. Results are variable and they cannot be recommended as a basic treatment for severe pain. Implantation carries the risk of infection but superficial stimulation is harmless and worth trying in difficult cases.

Hypnosis. It is well established that hypnosis may relieve pain in certain circumstances. The value of the technique in dentistry and obstetrics is accepted. Only a proportion of patients may be suitable subjects and hypnosis cannot be used for a planned procedure without previous assessment. In neurological medicine, the value of the technique is less well documented. It may be of value in relieving headache due to nervous tension and it is claimed to be helpful in intractable migraine where stress factors may be operative. There is no evidence that hypnosis has any useful effect on severe organic pain.

Acupuncture. Much recent interest has been aroused in this technique but the claims for acupuncture as a major analgesic technique have not yet been substantiated. Postherpetic neuralgia and severe sciatica appear to have been improved by acupuncture but why it should be is unknown. Manual or electrical vibration of the needle may act as a form of counter stimulation. The possibility of some form of hypnotic suggestion has also been raised. At the present time there is no established place for acupuncture in the relief of pain.

SPECIFIC PAIN PROBLEMS

Phantom Limb and Stump Pain. Phantom limb pain is distinct from the pain of an amputation stump. Stump pain is much commoner but the two types may coexist. Phantom pain is more usual when there has been severe trauma such as a crush injury to the amputated part.

Normally, a phantom diminishes in size so that the peripheral portion of the amputated part is in contact with the stump. Severe phantom limb pain is experienced only in about 5 per cent of patients. The pain is extremely difficult to treat. Cordotomy relieves the pain but will not alter the phantom and most patients learn to live with it. A destructive operation of the appropriate area of cerebral cortex may abolish the phantom but it is not recommended because the operation has to be extensive. Although cordotomy relieves phantom pain, the level of analgesia may recede and pain recur. In this case some improvement has been reported following posterior column stimulation.

Stump pain develops for several reasons. A painful stump scar may cause early pain and be eased by surgery. A stump neuroma develops after months or years and, again, often responds to surgical refashioning. An unsuitable prosthesis will cause pain and eventual ulceration of skin. However, despite these more obvious problems many patients continue to complain of pain. In some instances this is due to vascular insufficiency in the stump and may become worse as degenerative vascular disease is established.

Painful stumps can sometimes be helped by percussion therapy. A vibrator may also be used. In severe cases, especially when vascular factors are operative, a lumbar sympathectomy may be performed. Electrical stimulation of the stump is now being tried.

In the end, it may be necessary to resort to prescribing a combination of a phenothiazine and tricyclic antidepressant. This helps in the frequent situation where an affective component has emerged.

Postherpetic Neuralgia. This is common and unfortunately difficult to treat. Peripheral nerve section or chemical block is of no value. Patients do not usually report improvement on mild analgesics but one is reluctant to use more potent drugs in a non-malignant condition.

In spinal herpes zoster, anatomical lesions are usually present in the posterior root entry zone and even posterior nerve root section does not produce good results. The same objections apply to the intrathecal injection of phenol. It has been reported that CSF barbotage produces benefit but it is usually temporary. Attempts have been made to relieve the pain by excising and denervating the affected area of skin but it is not usually successful. The most effective surgical treatment is cordotomy. It is possible that dorsal column stimulation may prove helpful but it has not been established. Physical methods such as the use of a vibrator or ethyl chloride spray produce only temporary relief.

An affective component is an important feature in many patients with postherpetic neuralgia. Considerable success can be gained by using a combination of a phenothiazine and tricyclic antidepressant.

Causalgia. This is an extremely unpleasant burning pain that follows wounds of the nerves in the arms or legs. It was first described in detail in 1864 by Weir Mitchell, who gave the pain its present name. Causalgia is made worse by emotional disturbance and extremes of temperature. It is thought that there is a short-circuit of efferent sympathetic impulses to afferent conducting somatic fibres. In the upper limb, removal of the second and third cervical sympathetic ganglia relieves the burning pain but the increased sensitivity to temperature usually persists. Removal of the second and third lumbar ganglia may suffice for causalgia in the lower limb but if there is any question of involvement of the upper part of the sciatic nerve the first lumbar and twelfth thoracic ganglia should be removed.

Intercostal Neuralgia. Severe pain of a root distribution along the course of an intercostal nerve is a familiar and difficult problem. This may follow thoracotomy or a chest injury. It may be associated with dorsal spondylosis.

Section of the intercostal nerve does not usually relieve the pain. If the patient is stable emotionally the technique most likely to cure the pain is section of the posterior nerve roots. An initial anaesthetic block of the affected root and the one above and below should be carried out under radiological control. If success is obtained a laminectomy and section of the affected root and the two roots above and below should be carried out. The numbness that is felt is not of serious consequence.

6

Headache and Facial Pain

Many types of acute headache are discussed in other parts of this book. We are concerned here with the management of this common symptom and particularly the problem of recurrent and chronic headache.

In the assessment of headache a broad consideration of background psychological factors is particularly important, and these may be contributory even in cases where there is an organic basis for the pain. These factors cannot be identified in a brief and stereotyped interview, and demand a flexible approach. Two considerations stand out in discussions about non-specific headache. One is that headache may be localised to the site of a previous injury, often trivial, and sustained years before. It is hard to say whether the mechanism here is physical or psychological conditioning and both probably contribute. The second is the occurrence of headache after contact with a relative or associate with serious intracranial disease and the fear that a tumour is present. Sometimes several members of a family have developed a cerebral tumour and this reinforces anxiety. Rarely, such anxiety is well founded, and a tumour is demonstrated.

ACUTE HEADACHE AND FACIAL PAIN

When a local cause can be established, treatment is directed towards it. Acute sinusitis may require an antibiotic and measures to promote drainage. Acute iritis is relieved with local heat, analgesics, mydriatic, topical corticosteroid, and, when possible, treatment of the cause. Acute glaucoma is controlled with miotics, diuretics, and surgical measures. Dental pain requires local surgical treatment. In cervical spondylosis pain may be referred to the occipital region and responds to immobilisation with a collar.

Herpes Zoster Ophthalmicus. Pain may precede the appearance of the rash by several days, and sometimes persists afterwards for months or even years. The acute pain is of a shooting quality and may be aggravated by contact with the skin of the affected area. Pain may be controlled by local application of idoxuridine or systemic corticosteroid therapy (*see* page 233) and there is some evidence that this reduces the incidence of postherpetic neuralgia.

When *postherpetic neuralgia* is established, its management is usually difficult. Some cases respond to simple analgesics combined with chlorpromazine (75 to 600 mg daily) and an hypnotic such as dichloralphenazone or nitrazepam. In persistent cases counter-irritation with an electrical vibrator may help. An ethyl chloride spray will give temporary relief. The condition is commoner in the elderly and it may be thought justifiable to use more powerful analgesics such as pentazocine 200 mg or even morphine to ensure rest at night. Injection of the nerve and root section do not give relief and should be avoided.

If depression is a factor, imipramine or amitriptyline are worthwhile. Pericyazine 25 mg twice daily, later increased to from 60 to 90 mg daily is an alternative and can be used in combination with antidepressants. Occasionally, it may be thought appropriate to perform a surgical procedure to modify the appreciation of pain such as thalamotomy. Intrathecal ice-cold hypertonic saline may give relief but the effect is usually temporary.

Cranial Arteritis (giant cell arteritis: temporal arteritis). This disorder predominantly affects the elderly. Headache, pain on chewing, arthralgia, muscle pain (polymyalgia rheumatica) and fever may be present. In a typical case the temporal artery is tender and swollen. There may be sudden loss of vision due to infarction of the optic nerve. The erythrocyte sedimentation rate is high and the diagnosis may be confirmed by biopsy of an artery. It is a matter of urgency to start treatment in order to reduce the risk of loss of vision.

The treatment of choice is prednisolone and the initial dose 60 mg daily. This usually relieves headache and the other symptoms. After one to two weeks, if the symptoms and erythrocyte sedimentation rate are under control, the dose of prednisolone can be reduced to 30 mg daily, and after a further fortnight to 15 mg. This dose should be continued for at least six months and not withdrawn until the sedimentation rate is normal.

If a high dose of corticosteroid is needed to control the sedimentation rate, or steroid therapy is contra-indicated azathioprine may be given. The usual dose is 200 mg daily, and a careful check must be kept on the white cell count.

Trigeminal Neuralgia. Trigeminal neuralgia is a clinically distinct syndrome of facial pain. It usually arises around the mouth and may be triggered off by touching the face, eating, washing, or a cold wind. The pain is brief, excruciating, and recurrent. It may radiate to other parts of the face. It occurs in bouts that may last for a few weeks or longer. Severe trigeminal neuralgia may lead to weight loss and general debility.

The common type, seen mainly in elderly people, is not associated with physical signs, and its nature is obscure. The syndrome may be associated with brain stem disease such as multiple sclerosis or tumour and there are then likely to be signs of the underlying disease.

The pain often responds to carbamazepine 200 mg three times daily. The dose can be increased to 1200 mg daily or even 1800 mg. Regular administration is continued until the pain clears. The dose is then reduced to the minimum needed to control symptoms. Remission occurs after a variable time and relapse is common.

If relief is not obtained by drug therapy, surgical measures may be required. A branch of the nerve such as the infraorbital or supraorbital may be injected with alcohol or phenol. Avulsion of these nerves is occasionally carried out. Injection of the ganglion with alcohol (0·2 to 0·5 ml of 90 per cent) or phenol (0·5 ml of 5 per cent) is less selective but often relieves the pain. Stereotactic methods may be used to destroy the ganglion by applying heat or cold. Section of the nerve root is also employed and, occasionally, a tractotomy may be carried out. The results of these definitive treatments are good but some sensory loss over the face is produced. If the ophthalmic division is involved, there is risk of exposure keratitis. To prevent this, the eye may be protected with a shield or a tarsorrhaphy performed. Anaesthesia dolorosa is an occasional and troublesome sequel. Sometimes the symptoms recur in another division of the nerve.

Glossopharyngeal Neuralgia. Glossopharyngeal neuralgia is much less common than trigeminal neuralgia. The pain is of a similar type and provoked by swallowing. It may be located in the tongue or the region of the ear. Carbamazepine may give relief. The definitive treatment is section of the glossopharyngeal nerve in the posterior fossa, and it may be combined with section of the upper roots of the vagus nerve.

RECURRENT HEADACHE

Migraine. Migraine is a constitutional tendency to recurring headache associated with gastrointestinal upset, visual disturbances and other neurological deficits of a temporary kind. A family history is common. The mechanism is vascular; focal neurological features are attributed to vasoconstriction, and the headache to vasodilatation of the scalp vessels.

Many variants of the classical attack have been described. Partial or complete ophthalmoplegia may persist for days or even a few weeks (*ophthalmoplegic migraine*). The term *familial hemiplegic migraine* is usually reserved for those associated with dense hemiplegia which may be associated with aphasia and may last for many hours. Sometimes the pain is facial rather than cranial, a type known as *periodic migrainous neuralgia* or cluster headache. In one variety, a unilateral throbbing pain develops typically about 5 a.m. and is associated with lachrymation and unilateral nasal discharge. It clears after 30 minutes to a few hours, but tends to recur daily over a period of a few weeks or longer. After a remission it may return.

In the absence of physical signs between attacks, the investigation of patients with characteristic clinical histories by angiography and other methods is unhelpful and occasionally harmful.

Management can be considered under the headings of: (*a*) control of the acute attack; (*b*) interval therapy designed to reduce the number of attacks; and (*c*) general measures.

Acute Attack. Rest in a dark room followed by sleep gives relief. The most useful drug is ergotamine. Some attacks respond well to simple analgesics such as aspirin, compound codeine, dextroproxyphene 30 to 60 mg, dihydrocodeine tartrate 30 to 60 mg, indomethacin 25 to 50 mg, or perchlorperazine 5 to 10 mg.

Several routes of administration are possible with ergotamine tartrate. One milligram can be given by mouth or sublingually, but may aggravate nausea; 2 mg as a suppository is useful in resistant causes. An inhaler is suitable and, as a last resort, it can be given parenterally, but we do not recommend self-administration by this route (s.c. 0·5 mg; i.v. 0·25 mg). Ergotamine is most effective against headache when given during the aura.

Ergotamine tartrate should not be given during pregnancy. If it is used over a long period there is a minor risk of ergotism, and it is better avoided in patients with peripheral vascular disease. The safe limits for dosage are not known, but it is wise to avoid giving more than 6 mg in a period of 24 hours or more than 12 mg in a week. In severe, prolonged, and resistant cases it is reported that hydrocortisone 100 mg i.v. is useful, or dexamethasone 8 mg i.v. and either may be combined with intravenous ergotamine.

The most suitable therapy for patients with hemiplegia or other severe deficit presents difficulty. If ergotamine is used, the vasoconstrictor effect might aggravate the neurological deficit while giving relief of the headache.

Interval Therapy. Ergotamine is less useful as a prophylactic, and dihydroergotamine may be safer in a dosage of 1 mg three times daily, or up to 6 mg in 24 hours. It may be combined with sedation using nitrazepam at night.

Methysergide, an ergot derivative which is also a serotonin antagonist, is effective in about 60 per cent of cases if given in a dose of 3 to 6 mg daily over a period of weeks. Unfortunately, it has several unwanted effects, of which the most serious are fibrotic changes involving peritoneum, ureters, and other viscera. If retroperitoneal fibrosis develops it may progress even after the drug is stopped. We, therefore, advise that methysergide should be reserved for those with frequent, severe attacks and used in courses lasting up to six weeks.

Propranolol is of some value in prophylaxis. The dose is 20 mg twice daily at first and then increased in steps of 20 mg. It leads to bradycardia, hypotension, and cardiac failure if the dose is high, and also causes other effects due to blocking of beta adrenergic nerves.

Pizotifen is a serotonin antagonist which also has antihistamine actions. It is given in a dose of 0·5 mg three times daily and later increased to a maximum of 6 mg in 24 hours. It causes increase in appetite and drowsiness. Comparative trials show that it gives relief in about 50 per cent of patients, but it is not widely used. Clonidine is given in a dose of 25 to 75 μg daily, and helps some patients, although the benefits shown in controlled trials are less impressive.

Progesterone is worth considering in treating women with premenstrual migraine. The therapy is not established, and some workers consider that a fall in blood oestrogen level is a more important factor in provoking the headache.

Tricyclic antidepressants such as amitriptyline are useful. They will relieve depression, but there is evidence that 25 mg of amitriptyline given three times daily prevents migraine headache independently of its action in lifting mood.

The benzdiazopines; chlordiazepoxide (15 to 30 mg daily) and diazepam (6 to 15 mg daily) are useful as a supplementary therapy.

In summary, it may be said that clonidine may be helpful in milder cases. Methysergide, pizotifen, and propranolol are effective in a proportion of patients and may be used in sequence. When depression or anxiety are prominent, they may be supplemented with a benzdiazopine, or amitriptyline may be used alone. The assessment of drugs in the treatment of migraine presents many problems.

General Care. Patients are often referred to neurological clinics after a severe attack. Loss of speech is a particularly frightening event. Such people need an explanation of the nature of the disorder and reassurance that there is no progressive disease.

The contraceptive pill, and, notably, the oestrogen component may aggravate migraine, but this is variable from one patient to another. When attacks are aggravated, an alternative method of contraception is advised.

While sinus disease, infection elsewhere, and refractive errors may require treatment on their merits, there is no convincing evidence that the course of migraine is altered.

Persistence of a neurological deficit after an attack is rare and calls for a careful review of the diagnosis. The development of hypertension may aggravate migraine.

Blood Pressure and Headache. There is no simple relationship between headache and raised systemic blood pressure. Some patients with severe hypertension are free from headache. Others with severe hypertension report headache on waking in the morning, which clears in an hour or two. This type of headache is relieved when the blood pressure is controlled.

Headache in hypertensive patients may be a manifestation of anxiety about their blood pressure. This is upheld by the observation that headache is much less common in those who are unaware of their hypertension than in those who attend clinics for high blood pressure.

Headache and Cerebral Tumour. Although most patients with headache show no evidence of tumour, it is common for those with an intracranial tumour to develop headache. The type which is present on waking, and clears after an hour or two, is associated with raised intracranial pressure. Papilloedema is often found but may be absent. Headache of this type responds well to dexamethasone, but this drug should not be used until a policy of investigation and treatment has been decided. Pain may also be due to erosion of bone, as in pituitary tumour.

CHRONIC HEADACHE AND FACIAL PAIN

The patient who reports continuous headache over many years, and shows no physical signs is likely to have a chronic anxiety state, or depression. It is remarkable how often such patients have abandoned analgesic therapy, and indeed they respond poorly to it. *Atypical facial pain* may have a similar basis. Treatment is difficult. A sympathetic discussion of the life situation may help, and tranquillisers such as chlordiazepoxide and diazepam give some relief. Depression is an important factor, and treatment of it with drugs or physical methods will relieve headache. These therapies are discussed in Chapter 3.

When there is doubt whether a patient presents a psychological problem, it is wise to obtain a radiograph of the skull, and review the general medical condition. Temporo-mandibular dysfunction may cause persistent facial pain.

Among systemic medical disorders, three uncommon ones will be mentioned as they are easily overlooked. Chronic brucellosis is difficult to diagnose but may cause fever and headache. Paget's disease of the skull may be diagnosed clinically, or with a skull radiograph, and can cause severe and persistent headache which may respond to calcitonin therapy. Headache is commoner in patients with cerebral vascular disease than is generally recognised. In polycythaemia rubra vera, headache is a prominent feature.

The post-traumatic syndrome is discussed on pages 31 and 145.

7

Epilepsy

Epilepsy is a symptom, and the satisfactory management of any patient presenting with seizures depends on an assessment of the underlying cause. As the causes of epilepsy vary throughout life, the age of the patient is important. In childhood, birth trauma, neonatal infections and hereditary factors are significant. Subsequently, head injuries, cerebral tumours, and cerebrovascular disease become important.

Although there are several classifications of epilepsy, one helpful method is to try to decide whether attacks are primarily cortical or subcortical in origin. In primary subcortical (centrencephalic) epilepsy, generalised spike and wave discharges from 3 to 4½ Hz may be present on the EEG. Petit mal, idiopathic grand mal and certain types of myoclonic epilepsy are the corresponding clinical types. In cortical epilepsy, focal discharges are evident on the EEG in the area of the origin of the attack. Temporal lobe epilepsy is the commonest type of cortical epilepsy and has many clinical variants. Focal motor and sensory attacks are also relatively frequent. All of the focal clinical attacks may spread to produce a major seizure. A summary of the most important clinical types, related EEG abnormalities, and suitable drugs are shown in Table 7.1.

INVESTIGATION

The question of the degree to which one should investigate a patient with epilepsy is a matter of controversy. An adequate clinical description of the attack plus electroencephalography may be sufficient indication that the patient has subcortical epilepsy. On the other hand, the degree to which one should investigate someone presenting with cortical epilepsy is more difficult. This applies particularly with late onset epilepsy, which

Table 7.1
Classification of Epilepsy

Type	*Possible EEG abnormalities*	*Suitable drugs*
Petit mal (primary subcortical)	3–4½ Hz generalised spike and wave	ethosuximide sodium valproate troxidone
Grand mal (primary subcortical)	Interictal spike and wave	phenobarbitone phenytoin primidone carbamazepine sodium valproate
Myoclonic epilepsy (primary subcortical)	Polyspike and wave	nitrazepam clonazepam
Major seizures with cortical focus	Cortical foci + possible spike and wave	phenobarbitone phenytoin primidone carbamazepine sodium valproate
Focal motor attacks Focal sensory attacks	Cortical foci	phenytoin carbamazepine phenobarbitone primidone
Temporal lobe epilepsy	Temporal lobe	carbamazepine phenytoin primidone phenobarbitone
Infantile spasms	Gross multifocal spike and wave (Hypsarrhythmia)	corticotrophin nitrazepam clonazepam
Benign febrile convulsions	Normal	phenobarbitone (prophylactic) diazepam in acute attack

can be defined as epilepsy beginning after the age of twenty-five years. The object of investigating such patients is to ascertain whether there is a progressive focal lesion. Although one point of view is that the majority of patients with late onset epilepsy should be subjected to detailed neuroradiological investigation, this often does not help. In most instances, skull X-rays, and EEG and a brain scan should be sufficient to decide whether further investigations are necessary. Patients with slow-growing intracerebral gliomas may present with epilepsy that continues for several years without evidence of any positive neurological signs. It is doubtful whether the discovery of a glioma in someone presenting with epilepsy and no other disability is desirable. Many of these patients do very well for a number of years on anticonvulsant therapy. If they develop physical signs such as a facial weakness the time has come for further investigation. However, the advent of computerised transverse axial brain scanning has made the diagnosis of tumours possible at an early stage. The dilemma is that this diagnostic advance has outstripped the therapeutic capability to treat an infiltrating glioma.

An important point to bear in mind in the investigation of epilepsy, and indeed in the management of patients with epilepsy, is that the EEG although helpful on many occasions must not be regarded as a diagnostic computer. Many patients with epilepsy have a normal EEG and the diagnosis is a clinical one. It is not unknown for people to make a request to the EEG department for repeat EEGs, asking at the same time whether it is safe to stop anticonvulsants. The EEG has no place in providing such advice, and the decision must be based on clinical evidence.

DIFFERENTIAL DIAGNOSIS

Although epilepsy may frequently be easy to diagnose, there are instances when the diagnosis is uncertain, as for example when there is no adequate witness account of the attack, and where the patient is unable to provide any coherent history. Before coming to a definite conclusion it is necessary to wait on further events. It is unwise to treat epilepsy as such or apply a firm diagnostic label without adequate evidence. Hypoglycaemia may cause seizures in childhood and, less commonly, in adult life. An important cause of fits in adult life is the sudden withdrawal of drugs such as barbiturates. It is important to identify drug-induced fits and to distinguish them from true epilepsy.

Syncopal attacks may provide a problem and if prolonged may lead to convulsive movements. Another group is drop attacks. Drop attacks occur in teenage girls and middle-aged women. Some of these are emotional in origin. The patient drops to the ground without warning and there is difficulty in deciding whether there has been a brief lapse of consciousness. Many of these patients are labelled as akinetic epilepsy. In the younger age group this type of attack represents one type of hysterical fit. The florid and more obvious types of hysterical fits are more easily identified, particularly when one has the opportunity of witnessing them oneself. They may occur in the out-patient department or during EEG recording. In later life drop attacks may be due to vertebrobasilar disease, and sometimes a distinction between various types of focal epilepsy and migraine or transient ischaemic attacks is difficult. A repetitive stereotype nature of the attacks favours epilepsy. Patients with transient ischaemic attacks may have a less constant pattern of clinical presentation, and their attacks may last a good deal longer than could be expected with an ordinary focal epileptic seizure.

ANTICONVULSANT DRUGS

General Principles. The use of anticonvulsant drugs is of great importance in the management of the patient with epilepsy. Unfortunately, it is quite common to find that such drugs are misused. Some patients are suffering from drug toxicity and require much smaller doses of anticonvulsants to control their seizures. In other instances the combination of drugs is unsatisfactory and what could have been achieved with one or two drugs in appropriate dosage is achieved by a hotchpotch of medication that both the patient and doctor find confusing. A number of effective anticonvulsants are available and an adequate knowledge of their properties and side effects is essential in managing epilepsy.

Specific Anticonvulsants. The properties and pharmacological data covering the most important drugs are summarised in Table 7.2 but each drug is considered individually.

Phenobarbitone. This drug has been in use for many years and is still popular in the treatment of major and focal epilepsy. It is of no value in petit mal. The serum concentration correlates well with the oral dosage. The amount used varies from one clinician to another. High doses of phenobarbitone tend to cause drowsiness, depression, and impotence. In children there may be hyperkinetic behaviour disorders. Because the half-life of phenobarbitone is up to 140 hours, the drug can be given once or twice daily. We do not favour high doses because of side effects, and seldom use more than 120 mg daily. Phenobarbitone should be withdrawn slowly because of the risk of withdrawal fits. It should not be combined with primidone which is metabolised in part to phenobarbitone. Patients on long-term anticonvulsants may develop bilateral Dupuytren's contractures.

Phenytoin. This is a potent and widely used anticonvulsant. Proper use depends on adequate monitoring of serum levels. The drug is metabolised in the liver and only 5 per cent is excreted unchanged in the urine. There

Table 7.2. Summary of Clinical Pharmacology of Some Anticonvulsants

	Peak hours	*½-life hours*	*Complete excretion (days)*	*Therapeutic serum level mg/litre*	*Toxic serum level mg/litre*	*Dose mg/kg/day*	*Steady state*	*Enzyme induction*	*Terato-genic*	*Inter-actions*	*Dose frequency (daily)*
Phenytoin	4–8	10–17 up to 140 on treatment	3–5	10–20	15–30 rapid rise	9–13 ch 6–7 ad	5/10 days	Yes folate vit. D cortisol	Yes	protein binding state	1 or 2
Carbamazepine	2–5	8·5–19 after chronic treatment	does not accumulate	6–8	8–10	15–20	32 hr	Yes	less than others	lowers phenytoin levels	3
Phenobarbitone	6–18	37–73 ch 53–140 ad	10	15–25	30 tolerance	2–4	2/4 weeks	Yes vit. D etc.	Yes	lowers phenytoin levels	1
Primidone	3	3·3–12·5	8	5–10	10	9–15		Yes	Yes	lowers phenytoin levels	2
Ethosuximide	3	30 ch 60–100 ad.	10–15	40–80	?100	15–25	7 days	No	Not known		2
Sodium valproate	2	8–15	1	60–180		20–30 1200–2400 mg/day		No	In animals None yet in humans	potentiates all others, esp. seda-tive effect	3

Clonazepam	3	20–40		0·015–0·030		0·05–0·10	weeks	No	None yet	lowers phenytoin levels Develop tolerance	?1
Sulthiame	1–5	8	1–2	30				No	Not known	increases phenytoin levels	3

ch = child
ad = adult

is a wide variation in patient response. Doses ranging from 200 to 600 mg daily represents a usual range in the adult. Renal function deteriorating with age is one factor affecting tolerance. The rate of hepatic metabolism is under genetic control and varies in individuals. The addition of another drug that inhibits or induces phenytoin metabolism alters serum levels. Sulthiame inhibits metabolism and may precipitate toxicity. Carbamazepine induces metabolism and lowers the serum level of phenytoin. The therapeutic serum level of phenytoin is 10 to 20 mg/litre. At ranges above the figure quoted toxicity may not occur. A rapid rise in levels is more likely to precipitate toxicity.

The toxic effects of phenytoin are complex. Phenytoin intoxication may develop because the dose prescribed produces high serum levels in a person who metabolises the drug normally. In other instances the addition of other drugs such as sulthiame may precipitate toxicity. Some patients who have been stabilised on the same dose for some time develop intoxication without any change in therapy.

The acute cerebellar syndrome is characterised by ataxia, nystagmus, and dysarthria. Occasionally, there are hallucinations and in rare instances acute intoxication can be manifest as an abnormal mental state. The acute cerebellar syndrome responds to dose reduction in most cases. Sometimes ataxia persists and it has been suggested that phenytoin causes a fall out of Purkinje cells from the cerebellum. The evidence about this is in dispute. There may be an abnormal neuropsychiatric state and choreoathetosis.

Skin rash, lymphadenopathy, and, rarely, an LE syndrome may develop, and the drug should be withdrawn. Gingival hyperplasia and coarsening of the features is noted in many patients with therapeutic serum levels. A chronic peripheral neuropathy may develop in patients on long-term phenytoin the cause of which is unknown. Osteomalacia may be due to enzyme induction of vitamin D in the liver.

Folate deficiency is an established feature of long-term phenytoin therapy. Megaloblastic anaemia due to this deficiency responds to folic acid. However, the role of folate deficiency in the production of other unwanted effects is a matter of dispute. There is no direct evidence that it is involved in the side effects already mentioned. It has been suggested that some patients who develop a chronic neuropsychiatric disturbance while on phenytoin do respond to folic acid although this may be associated with an increased frequency of seizures. The work is not universally accepted and the precise role of folate metabolism in the anticonvulsant action of phenytoin is unknown.

Phenytoin has been incriminated in the production of fetal abnormalities. There is no clear-cut evidence on this complex point. The treatment of epilepsy must still take precedence in pregnancy. Mothers on anticonvulsants may still breast feed as the concentration of phenytoin in milk is insignificant.

Primidone. The metabolites of primidone are active anticonvulsants. Primidone is similar in structure to phenobarbitone and is converted to phenylethylmalonamide and phenobarbitone. The therapeutic effect to a large extent is due to the latter metabolite. The serum concentration of primidone is at least half that of phenobarbitone but similar to phenylethylmalonamide. The half-life of phenobarbitone is much longer than primidone. The two drugs should not be given in combination.

The more important side effects of primidone are an acute ataxic disorder with vertigo and mental confusion, depression, loss of libido, drowsiness, skin rashes, folate deficiency, and megaloblastic anaemia. An aplastic anaemia has been reported on rare occasions.

Carbamazepine. Evidence is accumulating that this is an anticonvulsant of value in major seizures and temporal lobe epilepsy. It is chemically related to the tricyclic antidepressants and is effective in elevating mood and improving behavioural problems in patients with epilepsy. Routine serum levels are not generally available. The drug may cause skin rashes, gastrointestinal disturbance, vertigo and ataxia, and occasionally leucopenia and marrow aplasia. Hepatic damage has been reported. The side effects of carbamazepine have been exaggerated. It is a useful anticonvulsant.

Ethosuximide. This is the drug of choice in petit mal. Two metabolites are produced via hepatic breakdown. Serum levels of the drug have been measured but they are not routinely available. However, studies show that the serum concentration is related to the efficacy of the drug and adequate control of petit mal may be achieved at 40 to 120 mg/litre. Ethosuximide is the most effective of the succinamide group of drugs. There are few side effects. Occasionally, nausea and drowsiness occur. Leucopenia has been recorded.

Troxidone. The need for this drug is infrequent. Less toxic and more effective preparations are available for petit mal. The therapeutic activity is due to dimethadione. Troxidone may cause bone marrow depression and a visual glare phenomenon.

Sodium Valproate. Complete assessment of this drug is not yet possible. Controlled studies have shown it has anticonvulsant properties in petit mal and major attacks. It is unrelated to other anticonvulsants. Side effects include, nausea, vomiting, and drowsiness.

Benzodiazepines. Diazepam is established as an effective intravenous therapy for status epilepticus. It is relatively ineffective as an oral anticonvulsant. Nitrazepam has been used as an oral agent in myoclonic seizures and petit mal with some success. The most recent drug introduced in this group is clonazepam. Trials have suggested it is effective in petit mal, myoclonic epilepsy, and in major and minor seizures. Drowsiness has proved a troublesome side effect and the dose schedule can be difficult to establish. Clonazepam is effective in status epilepticus but the intravenous preparations must be freshly prepared using two ampoules. Clonazepam has yet to be fully assessed.

Sulthiame. Unfortunately, there is no evidence to support worthwhile independent activity of this drug. It has been widely used but its main effect is as an inhibitor of phenobarbitone, primidone, and phenytoin metabolism. Drug intoxication is frequently precipitated. In addition, hyperventilation and psychotic states occur. It is related to the sulphonamides. On present evidence there is no reason for using it.

Pheneturide. This is an acetylurea compound. No proper trial has ever been performed with it using a placebo. The drug inhibits the metabolism of phenytoin and phenobarbitone and produces drowsiness and ataxia. It is of doubtful value.

Beclamide. Little use is now made of this drug. It has been claimed to have a stimulant effect and to improve behaviour. It was used in retarded disturbed patients with epilepsy. There is very little evidence to support its continuing use.

Chlormethiazole. There is no evidence of oral anticonvulsant activity but an intravenous preparation has been used successfully in status epilepticus. It has no advantage over clonazepam or diazepam.

TREATMENT

General Considerations. Once a diagnosis of epilepsy is established and a rational approach to any underlying cause is determined, the question of appropriate drug treatment is foremost. A single fit in an adult does not constitute a diagnosis of epilepsy. Although some would advocate drug therapy for a single seizure in an adult, we recommend withholding therapy to await subsequent events. A single fit may herald a tumour but there is little to be lost in delaying therapy until the need for continuous treatment is firmly established. The choice of drug depends to some extent on the type of attack and age of the patient. It is important to adopt a clear policy on follow-up of patients on anticonvulsants. There are few special clinics for epilepsy in existence and most patients are seen in general practice or hospital out-patients. The repeat prescription system in general practice leads to inadequate supervision, and patients on anticonvulsants should be regularly seen by their general practitioner even if they are under hospital supervision.

The development of techniques for estimating serum levels of anticonvulsants has proved valuable in controlling patients on phenytoin and, to a lesser extent, phenobarbitone. In the future, estimation of serum levels of other anticonvulsants may have a place in the management but this is not yet established.

Drug interactions in patients on anticonvulsants have assumed increasing importance. This applies to the interaction between different anticonvulsants and changes that take place as a result of taking anticonvulsants in relation to drugs used for general medical disease.

Inhibition of anticonvulsant metabolism by competition in the same metabolic pathway or enzyme inhibition will increase serum levels of the relevant anticonvulsant. Sulthiame inhibits phenytoin, phenobarbitone and primidone metabolism and thus raises their serum levels. Pheneturide also increases phenytoin and phenobarbitone serum levels.

Induction, which accelerates drug metabolism, may develop when benzodiazepines are added to phenytoin. However, this is probably of little clinical significance. Carbamazepine reduces serum phenytoin levels and the administration of folic acid has a similar effect.

With regard to drugs in general medical use, anticonvulsants reduce the dose of warfarin required and steroid hormone metabolism is induced.

EPILEPSY IN CHILDHOOD

Convulsions in Infancy. Neonatal convulsions cause death or serious brain damage unless rapidly controlled. Underlying biochemical disturbances are frequently relevant. Hypoglycaemia, hypomagnesaemia, hypocalcaemia, or pyridoxine deficiency may require correction. Therapeutic trials of the various agents is recommended, preferably after blood level estimations. A therapeutic trial of pyridoxine is always worthwhile. If the cause is acute infection such as *Escherichia coli* meningitis, specific treatment must be given for this as well as the seizures. In the case of repeated seizures, diazepam up to 1 mg/kg or more may be used. For prophylaxis of neonatal convulsions due to brain damage, phenobarbitone is the most effective drug, maintaining a serum level of around 10 to 20 mg/litre. In practice, this involves 45 to 75 mg daily.

Infantile spasms have a variety of causes. Clinically, they are manifested by 'jack knife' attacks or salaam spasms. They may be associated with tuberose sclerosis or follow pertussis immunisation. Adenocorticotrophic hormone (ACTH) has been recommended as the treatment of choice. The spasms are often associated with mental retardation. The dose of ACTH is empirical, and although early improvement is reported the long-term results with regard to mental development and seizure control are disappointing.

The end result depends on the widely differing underlying causes for the spasms. Despite this, ACTH is usually given in a dose of 20 to 30 units for three to four weeks. Benzodiazepines, notably nitrazepam and clonazepam, have been used alone or in conjunction with ACTH in infantile spasms. The long-term benefits of these is as uncertain as it is with ACTH. Nitrazepam should be given in a dose of 1 mg/kg/day.

Febrile convulsions occurring from six months to five years but usually between the ages of two and five are no longer regarded as benign since it has been shown that a prolonged febrile convulsion might lead to temporal lobe epilepsy in later life. The recurrence rate after a single convulsion is about 45 per cent. The treatment involves that of the acute attack and the controversial matter of prophylaxis up to the age of five.

In the acute attack the convulsion is best controlled with diazepam and the temperature lowered with aspirin, ice packs, and tepid sponging. Antibiotics should be given if there is a primary bacterial infection.

Prophylaxis using phenytoin has proved unsuccessful and intermittent phenobarbitone at the time of the fever is of no value. A trial of continuous phenobarbitone in the doses mentioned above to maintain a level of 10 to 20 mg/litre has been shown to be effective. Currently we recommend the use of phenobarbitone prophylaxis after a prolonged convulsion or where focal neurological features are present.

Petit Mal. This is primarily a condition of children and rarely presents a problem in adult life. The common age of onset is around five years. Troxidone was the first drug to be used with success but has now been superseded by ethosuximide, the most effective of the succinamide group. The dose required to control absence attacks may be up to 1500 to 2000 mg daily in divided doses. A plasma level of 40 mg/litre appears to be the minimum required to control attacks. A dose of 20 mg/kg body weight is an average dose.

Benzodiazepines have been used in petit mal but their efficacy is uncertain and they are not superior to ethosuximide. Nitrazepam, clonazepam, and diazepam are effective in controlling petit mal status. In routine treatment their place has not been established. The hypnotic effects of clonazepam have limited its use. With a starting dose of 0·25 mg at night and gradually increasing to 2 mg a day improvement may be seen. Sodium valproate is effective in petit mal but has been introduced too recently for its final evaluation. It has fewer side effects than clonazepam, and 800 to 2000 mg daily may be required.

MYOCLONIC EPILEPSY

Myoclonus is the brief and rapid involuntary jerking of muscles. It is frequently bilateral and proximal. Myoclonic jerks may be a feature of patients with primary subcortical epilepsy who develop brief jerkings of the limbs, mainly in the early morning. Myoclonic jerking may be associated with petit mal absence attacks. There is also a form of benign essential myoclonic epilepsy that takes place throughout life and is not associated with loss of consciousness. This may run in families.

Myoclonus is also a feature of serious progressive disorders of the nervous system. The jerks seen in infantile spasms are myoclonic, and myoclonic jerking may also occur in the lipidoses, subacute sclerosing panencephalitis, and the Jakob-Creutzfeldt syndrome. Rare types of progressive myoclonic epilepsy are described with dementia, and the presence of Lafora amyloid inclusion bodies within the nervous system. Myoclonus may also be a feature of cerebellaris dyssynergia myoclonica, a progressive form of cerebellar degeneration. Occasionally, segmental myoclonus is due to spinal disease.

Myoclonic petit mal may respond to ethosuximide or sodium valproate. Nitrazepam 1 mg/kg/day is also effective in benign types of myoclonic epilepsy and may be of value in infantile spasms. Clonazepam is likely to be as effective as nitrazepam and is now being more widely used. The prognosis in the more serious diseases associated with myoclonus is poor, and drugs are of limited value.

REFLEX EPILEPSY

A number of rare types of reflex epilepsy such as musicogenic and reading epilepsy are treated with anticonvulsants. The commonest variety is photic epilepsy induced by a flickering television set or the flashing lights in a discotheque. The EEG commonly shows a photoconvulsive response with spike and wave discharges to flashes of light commonly at 15 to 20 Hz.

There may be a positive photic response in patients with primary subcortical epilepsy, but in their case attacks take place at other times and the resting record is often abnormal. A photoconvulsive response should not be confused with a photomyoclonic response. In the latter, the EEG discharge and the myoclonic jerks stop when the stimulus is removed.

Photic epilepsy can be prevented by avoiding the flickering light or covering one eye. This is preferable to anticonvulsant therapy.

EPILEPSY IN ADULTS

Major Seizures. On present evidence the primary drugs are still phenobarbitone, phenytoin, primidone and, more recently, carbamazepine.

Phenobarbitone may be used in a dose of 90 mg daily. It may be given as a single dose, a dose of more than 120 mg generally causing mental slowing, loss of libido, and depression. Phenobarbitone must be withdrawn gradually because of its long half-life.

Phenytoin in a dose from 200 to 600 mg daily may be used in addition to phenobarbitone or alone. The ideal is to control the patient on one drug. In practice, phenytoin is more effective. Serum levels of phenytoin are required if side effects develop or control is unsatisfactory.

Primidone must not be combined with phenobarbitone. It may cause an acute toxic reaction on as little as 125 mg. The dose may range from 250 to 1500 mg daily but on the higher doses somnolence and ataxia may ensue. Primidone and phenytoin may be used together.

Carbamazepine is increasingly used. The dose may range from 400 mg to 2 g daily. Unsteadiness and vertigo may occur on the higher doses. The authors regard carbamazepine as preferable to primidone and it can be regarded, with phenytoin, as a potent anticonvulsant in major attacks.

The newer anticonvulsants are of less importance. Sodium valproate may prove valuable in major attacks. Sulthiame, pheneturide, and beclamide have no established place in treatment.

With care in choosing the most useful drug and dose, the majority of patients with major seizures may obtain good control. Regular observation and attention to general care and problems are important.

Focal Seizures. There is no evidence to support the superiority of any of the above drugs in focal motor or sensory attacks. Ethosuximide is of no value in minor temporal lobe seizures. In temporal lobe epilepsy primidone has been suggested as first choice. Recent studies suggest that carbamazepine is the only drug that may be more effective and we regard it as the drug of choice in temporal lobe attacks. The dose may range from 400 mg to over 2000 mg a day; 100 and 200 mg tablets are available. The dose may have to be pushed to a high level to obtain good control of minor temporal lobe attacks. In doing this the disadvantages of high dose therapy must be considered, for some people with temporal lobe epilepsy are not unduly bothered by brief attacks and prefer to take little or no treatment. One should not strive to control attacks at the expense of the patient's well being.

STATUS EPILEPTICUS

The treatment of this emergency has improved considerably, but the mortality is still approximately 20 per cent. The difference between serial epilepsy and status epilepticus is one of degree. The general practitioner is the first on the scene. If possible, he is best advised to give 10 mg of diazepam intravenously or intramuscularly. Paraldehyde by intramuscular injection is probably better than diazepam by the same route.

Status epilepticus must be stopped quickly to prevent serious brain damage. Hyperpyrexia needs controlling with tepid sponging or ice packs.

The current drugs of choice are diazepam and clonazepam. Diazepam is simpler to use as clonazepam powder needs to be made into a fresh solution at the time of use. Diazepam, 10 mg intravenously over two minutes usually controls status but recurrence is frequent. The dose may be repeated, but with further relapses 100 mg in 500 ml of normal saline may be infused over twelve hours. There may be hypotension and respiratory depression. Clonazepam is ten times more potent weight for weight than diazepam. An initial dose of 2 mg intravenously may be given, or an infusion of 8 to 10 mg in 500 ml of 5 per cent dextrose over twelve hours.

Barbiturates either short or long acting have been used in status epilepticus. Thiopentone is the most effective short acting drug in a dose of 150 to 200 mg. The dose required is usually less than that required to produce anaesthesia. Phenobarbitone does not act quickly and repeated doses lead to respiratory depression.

Phenytoin also acts slowly. An intravenous injection of 500 to 1000 mg may be given at the time of initial control, and the drug continued in a dose of 300 mg orally or intravenously each day. Paraldehyde will control status but it acts slowly. It dissolves plastic syringes and has an unpleasant smell. It may be given intravenously in a dose of 3·5 ml in saline but has no advantage over diazepam or clonazepam.

If the fits continue, it may be necessary to curarise the patient and use positive pressure respiration (page 10). This does not remove the need for anticonvulsants.

When managing status epilepticus, it is important not to withdraw parenteral therapy too soon, but at the same time the patient should be established on a long-term anticonvulsant regime; phenytoin is the most useful drug. Status often results from irregular therapy but some individuals are particularly prone to it and this grave complication may supervene in someone previously seizure-free.

SURGERY OF EPILEPSY

Only a very small number of patients with epilepsy are suitable for surgical treatment. No patient with epilepsy should be subjected to surgery without a prolonged course of medical treatment in expert hands. The majority of patients with epilepsy who have surgical operations have temporal lobe epilepsy. They are best operated on in special centres that have wide experience of this type of operation. There seems little doubt that in selected cases and in suitable hands, anterior temporal lobectomy can reduce seizure frequency and, sometimes, abolish seizures in patients with intractable temporal lobe epilepsy. The place of surgical treatment in other types of epilepsy is less well defined. Attempts may be made to remove a clear-cut focus in a region other than the temporal lobe but these operative ventures are frequently associated with failure, and extreme caution should be exercised before subjecting a patient to such procedures. Other operative approaches such as section of the corpus callosum, and hemispherectomy for infantile hemiplegia associated with intractable epilepsy may occasionally have a place in the management of a difficult patient. However, the place of surgery in epilepsy should be put into perspective and it is only a minority of patients who are suitable for any sort of surgical procedure at the present time. It seems unlikely that surgery will have any greater place in the treatment of epilepsy in the future.

SOCIAL ASPECTS OF EPILEPSY

The social implications of having epilepsy are rather different in children and adults. Unfortunately, it is still true that many members of the general population regard the fact that someone has epilepsy as a stigma. There is still need for education of the general public on this subject. It is not uncommon to encounter difficulties with employers and school authorities.

Childhood. In children, many of the difficulties relate to schooling and the social restrictions that may be imposed upon the child. A number of children with epilepsy naturally have additional handicaps that may be far more important than the actual epileptic attacks. If the child is educationally subnormal, special provisions will have to be made for schooling. However, many children whose attacks are infrequent can be educated at a normal school, do perfectly satisfactory work, and enter into school activities. Sometimes great difficulty is encountered in persuading school authorities that a child should continue to go to school although having some attacks. The child may be sent home and not be allowed to return to school until perfect control is achieved. The attitude about this varies considerably from area to area and from school to school and undoubtedly some schools find it much more difficult than others to cope with the problem child with epilepsy. Normally, children with epilepsy should not be kept off school unless the attacks are frequent and impossible to deal with. Unfortunately, children who do have epilepsy are often told that they must not take part in school games of any kind, nor must they go swimming. In our opinion, children with epilepsy that is controlled, should be allowed to play ball games and enter into athletic activities, although they should not climb wall bars or ladders. It is reasonable to allow the child to go swimming when accompanied by a responsible adult. A tolerant attitude does prevent a great deal of the social isolation that will otherwise occur. It is important if the child is taking drugs several times a day that adequate provision is made for them to be taken during school hours. Children should not be left to their own devices with regard to drug taking because they frequently omit their medication.

In some instances the frequency of attacks and other problems will require a child to be sent to a special school for children with epilepsy. In approved cases local authorities apply for places to be provided at the special schools. In children meriting this form of education great benefit can be obtained. The most important problem is to recognise the educational requirements at an early age so that appropriate application can be made.

Adolescents with frequent attacks often find it difficult to form adequate social relationships and they may become extremely lonely. Even though they may be encouraged to join youth clubs or enter other activities they become isolated and are not fully integrated with friends of their own age. The attitude and role that the parents take in this type of difficulty is most important. There is only a limited amount the doctor or social worker can achieve. Sometimes the original difficulty arises from the parents being over-protective, and this should be avoided.

Secondary behaviour disorders and other psychiatric disturbances do develop in children with epilepsy but the term 'epileptic personality' should not be used. Most of the behavioural disturbances that exist arise from difficulties outlined above or are related to additional organic brain disease or to the drug treatment the child has been given.

Adults. In adults the difficulties that arise in the social field are different, although they may have lacked satisfactory education as a result of epilepsy in childhood. At the time of leaving school many young adults have difficulty in gaining employment, particularly in areas where unemployment is high. Sometimes, although they may undergo training schemes, there is difficulty in finding sympathetic employers, although, of course, large firms are compelled to take a small percentage of registered disabled persons. There are many types of employment patients with epilepsy are quite suitable to undertake and there is a lot of mythology surrounding the question of safety at work. Much modern machinery is well guarded and there is virtually no risk of a patient who has an attack doing himself any harm. Naturally there are jobs that involve climbing or handling dangerous materials, and these are quite unsuitable. One serious problem that may occur is when a man who is well established in his work develops epilepsy in adult life and his promotion prospects, and even his job, are jeopardised. This may be because driving is an integral part of the job and the patient has to be told to stop driving, advice that may not be accepted by the patient.

Epilepsy and Driving. The present law (United Kingdom) about driving and epilepsy states that a patient must be free of attacks for a period of at least three years with or without treatment. The only exception to this rule is patients with nocturnal epilepsy whose attacks have been solely nocturnal for a period of over three years. A single fit after the age of three years precludes the holding of heavy goods vehicle licence. It is most important to give appropriate advice on the question of driving and to put it in writing. This is sometimes difficult and the patient may take offence at the suggestion. If he does not take advice about stopping driving because of epilepsy, the physician is placed in a difficult position. He could be regarded as breaching the ethic of patient confidence by reporting the epilepsy to the licensing authority. However, it is the doctor's duty to do this if he knows that a patient, when he is told to stop driving, is continuing to do so.

Anticonvulsants should not be reduced or stopped after a three-year period of freedom if driving is to be re-started.

Marriage. Sometimes epilepsy places very considerable strains on a marriage relationship, particularly when the attacks are frequent or have occurred after the marriage has started. If there is a disturbance in sexual relationships the stress may be even greater. Epilepsy may be associated with impotence and reduced libido and this is particularly so with regard to temporal lobe epilepsy. Epilepsy existing prior to marriage and undeclared, is a ground for annullment of the marriage in England.

Women with epilepsy often have problems in the house and in the general management of their children which gives them cause for concern. In many instances they can be reassured. Some younger mothers are worried that they may drop their children when nursing them at an early age. This can happen, but it is rare. If a woman with severe epilepsy does have a young family she will require some sort of help in the management of her children but normally such severely disabled mothers are advised to avoid pregnancy. Advice is often requested about the relationship between pregnancy and an increase in the frequency of attacks, and also the advisability of using the oral contraceptive pill. Some patients with epilepsy who are pregnant have no problems. In other instances there is an increase in the frequency of attacks. Pregnancy, therefore, has a variable influence on the course of the condition. With regard to the pill there is no definite evidence that the pill increases the frequency of epilepsy, although in some instances this may appear to be so. If there is sufficient evidence to confirm increased frequency the oral contraceptive should be stopped.

Heredity. The question of heredity in epilepsy is a matter of common concern. There is frequently a fear that if a man or woman has the condition then their children may be affected. The best advice to give in these circumstances is that although epilepsy can appear in more than one generation, it is not inherited in a clear-cut manner. Patients with primary subcortical epilepsy are more likely to pass on the condition to their relatives than those with other types of epilepsy. Primary subcortical epilepsy is probably inherited as a mendelian dominant with variable penetrance. It should be explained that there is a greater likelihood of epilepsy appearing when there is one member affected in a family, but this is a small risk, and general reassurance may be given. It is undesirable for two people with a family history of epilepsy to marry.

Institutions. The majority of patients with epilepsy are able to maintain an independent existence. Even if they are not, many of them are looked after in their home environment. However, situations do exist where patients with epilepsy cannot be looked after at home, and these patients may require admission to a special centre, a number of which exist throughout the UK. In the past they used to be called Epileptic Colonies, a term that is no longer acceptable. These centres not only look after the patients with particularly severe epilepsy, trying to give them as normal an environment as possible, but they also have shorter-stay units where difficult problems can be assessed and where the patient may be sent for detailed assessment and for improved management. It is likely that such centres will increase in number in the future.

Deviant Behaviour. Occasionally, patients with epilepsy commit antisocial or criminal acts as a result of their attacks. This is much rarer than is generally believed. It is true that sexual misdemeanours or other criminal acts may be committed in a state of postepileptic automatism, but it is more frequent for the patient to use his attacks as an excuse for his behaviour. Great care should therefore be used in analysing all the factors involved if requested to make a judgement on whether a patient's behaviour has resulted from his epilepsy.

NARCOLEPSY

Narcolepsy may occur as an isolated symptom of excessive hypersomnia, or form part of a symptom complex. The associated disturbances are sleep paralysis, cataplexy, and hypnagogic hallucinations. Isolated narcolepsy must be distinguished from other causes of hypersomnia, which include hypothalamic tumours, cardiorespiratory syndrome associated with obesity, encephalitis, endogenous depression, and the action of sedative drugs.

Narcolepsy responds to treatment with dextroamphetamine 10 to 60 mg daily in divided doses. The last dose should not be given after 4.00 p.m. Combination with clomipramine or desipramine may reduce the amphetamine requirements. Clomipramine has some beneficial effect on cataplexy and hypnagogic hallucinations. It is seldom necessary to use more than 75 mg daily. Narcolepsy is the main indication for the use of amphetamine in current medical practice. Tolerance is uncommon when it is used in this group of disorders.

8

Parkinsonism and Involuntary Movement

PARKINSONISM

Parkinsonism provides a good example of a common neurological disorder for which effective therapy can be provided despite almost complete ignorance of the aetiology.

The onset is usually insidious and the features are often not recognised by those who are in close contact with the patient. The exact incidence is unknown but the prevalence has been estimated at one per thousand. The disease is uncommon below the age of 50 years, and increases in incidence with age. In the majority of cases the cause remains unknown, and this chapter is primarily concerned with the management of this form of the disease.

Pathological Physiology. Parkinsonism is associated with changes in the basal ganglia. In the postencephalitic form a characteristic feature is loss of pigment from the substantia nigra. The histology of this area and the pallidum shows destruction and fall-out of neurones containing melanin. Similar changes are found in the common variety of Parkinsonism. The advances in treatment have come from study of the biochemistry of amines, and the effect of lesions in structures that connect with the basal ganglia.

Interest in the amine content of the brain began about twenty years ago when it was shown that the administration of reserpine to man or animals could lead to a Parkinsonian syndrome. This was reversed by withdrawal of the drug or the administration of dopa. The next major step was the demonstration by histochemical methods that the normal striatum and substantia nigra contain high concentrations of dopamine and that this is reduced in animals treated with reserpine, and in patients with Parkinsonism.

Dopamine does not pass the blood-brain barrier, and for clinical purposes levodopa is administered by mouth and is converted to dopamine in the brain. Dopamine is broken down by the enzyme dopa decarboxylase, which is widely distributed in the body. Recent work has been directed towards the use of inhibitors of dopa decarboxylase, and two of these—carbidopa and benserazide—are now in general use. Carbidopa and benserazide are not effective when given alone.

Diagnosis. The diagnosis of Parkinsonism is clinical and can often be made as soon as the patient is seen, particularly if he is observed when walking, and does not swing the arms. The clinical features can be grouped under the headings hypokinesia, rigidity, tremor, and loss of associated movements. *Hypokinesia* implies a delay in the initiation of movement, with slowness, restriction, and impairment of motor function, including speech. There is no diagnostic laboratory test, although the level of homovanillic acid (derived from dopamine) in spinal fluid is usually reduced in patients with Parkinsonism.

The tremor of Parkinsonism must be distinguished from essential tremor which effects mainly the arms and head, is more rapid, evolves very slowly, and is often familial. There may be hypokinetic features in depression. Patients with systemic neurological diseases, of which Parkinsonism forms a component, such as the Shy-Drager syndrome, and progressive supranuclear palsy may not respond well to levodopa.

THERAPEUTIC MEASURES

There is no evidence that the therapy currently available has any influence on the pathological process in the basal ganglia. The mere presence of Parkinsonism is not, in itself, an indication for any therapy. The unwanted effects of the various drugs are frequent enough to justify withholding them when symptoms are minimal.

Treatment of the cause is seldom possible. Arteriosclerosis is common in patients with Parkinsonism, but it is doubtful whether it is a significant factor, although infarction of the basal ganglia may contribute in some cases. Encephalitis lethargica, a presumed virus disease, is now uncommon, but patients who survived the earlier epidemics are sometimes seen. Poisoning with carbon monoxide or manganese can produce a Parkinsonian syndrome. Wilson's disease must always be considered in the child or adult under 40, and the clinical diagnosis is clinched by finding a deposit of copper in the cornea (Kayser-Fleischer ring). In many patients the initial clinical manifestations of Parkinsonism are unilateral, and later become bilateral. This may raise the possibility of a tumour, but it is rare. Head injury seldom causes Parkinsonism, probably because most patients with injury to the basal ganglia do not survive, but it may be a feature of the punch drunk syndrome of boxers.

Drug Therapy. There can be no doubt that the introduction of levodopa has been the major advance in therapy. Levodopa is less toxic than its stereoisomers, but unwanted effects are troublesome and in the long term about 50 per cent of patients are helped by this drug.

While tremor is an embarrassment to the patient and weakness is not a feature of the disease, it has recently become clear that the main motor disability is due to *hypokinesia.* The effect of levodopa is most striking in reducing hypokinesia. It also eases rigidity, and some patients find improvement in tremor. Difficulty in carrying out fine movements, immobility of facial expression, and dribbling of saliva (due to impaired swallowing) may all be relieved.

Levodopa is given by mouth, but commonly causes anorexia and nausea. The combination of levodopa with a dopa decarboxylase inhibitor reduces the gastric effects. Treatment can be started with 125 mg levodopa + 12·5 mg carbidopa or 100 mg levodopa + 25 mg benserazine twice daily. After two days the dose can be doubled and later increased further if necessary. In most patients a response is obtained by the time the daily dosage reaches 500 to 1000 mg levodopa with 50 to 100 mg carbidopa, or 400 to 800 mg levodopa with 100 to 200 mg benserazine.

The equivalent dosages are—

1 g levodopa = 250 mg levodopa + 25 mg carbidopa (Sinemet)
= 200 mg levodopa + 50 mg benserazine (Madopar)

If one pair of drugs fails it is worth trying the other.

It would now seem that there is little place for levodopa alone. If it is given, the initial dose is 250 mg twice daily, and after a week it is increased to 500 mg twice daily. Further increase in steps of 250 mg at intervals of five days is usually tolerated. Nausea may be relieved by giving metoclopramide 10 to 30 mg with each dose.

Some patients develop dizziness, light-headedness, confusion, insomnia, delirium, or hypotension, and these may be limiting factors in dosage. Levodopa is not well tolerated by patients with postencephalitic Parkinsonism, and they are prone to develop psychosis. Pre-existing psychosis of any kind may be aggravated.

Preparations containing levodopa should not be used in combination with monoamine oxidase inhibitors, but levodopa is compatible with tricyclic antidepressants. Glaucoma may be aggravated. Levodopa in large doses may aggravate cardiac arrhythmias, and is antagonised by pyridoxine.

The main unwanted effect in the long term is the development of *involuntary movements* (dyskinesia). They are commonly choreiform and affect the face, fingers, and toes. Occasionally, they are gross. They tend to appear after several years of treatment, but may come on early. High dosage may provoke involuntary movements at any stage. Mild involuntary movements may be tolerated, but when troublesome can be relieved only by reducing the dose. Adjustment of the frequency of dosage may help.

There may be fluctuations in the disability even in the untreated Parkinsonian patient. Sometimes there is deterioration two to four hours after levodopa has been given, and this may be offset by more frequent dosage. Some patients show abrupt swings from akinesia to almost normal movement, which is termed the on/off phenomenon. Management is difficult. Adjustment of dosage and frequency of administration may help, and withdrawal of the drug followed by reintroducing it in lower dosage a few weeks later is worthwhile.

Persistent involuntary movement or psychotic change may make it necessary to withdraw levodopa therapy. No serious long-term effects have so far been reported.

Amantadine. This drug was introduced as an antiviral agent, and shown to be of benefit in Parkinsonism. The usual dose is 100 mg twice daily, and may be increased to 400 mg daily if tolerated. There are no serious toxic effects, but ankle oedema and livedo reticularis may occur. High doses may cause hallucinations. It is much less potent than levodopa, but may relieve rigidity and hypokinesia. The effect tends to diminish over a period of weeks. The mode of action is uncertain. A response to amantadine is of no help in predicting whether a patient will respond well to levodopa.

Anticholinergic Drugs. Hyoscine and atropine have been used for many years. They relieve rigidity, as may be shown dramatically when a patient who has been taking a regular dose suddenly stops and 'freezes'. The drugs in common use are listed in Table 8.1, and benzhexol is often preferred. They may cause dryness of the mouth, constipation, blurred vision, and confusion. If the dose is increased slowly, surprisingly large amounts may be tolerated, and are particularly useful in postencephalitic Parkinsonism. Anticholinergic drugs can be used in combination with levodopa or amantadine.

Table 8.1. Anticholinergic Drugs

Drug	*Proprietary name*	*Daily dose (mg)*	*Frequency of dose*	*Unwanted effects*
Benzhexol	Artane	4–30	3/day	dry mouth
Benztropine	Cogentin	1–5	at night	constipation blurred vision
Orphenadrine	Disipal	150 +	3/day	confusional state
Procyclidine	Kemadrin	2·5 to 10	3/day	aggravates glaucoma retention of urine

Combined Drug Therapy and General Application. In mild cases of Parkinsonism, particularly in the elderly, benzhexol is useful and can be combined with amantadine. Where hypokinesia is prominent levodopa is the drug of choice. Levodopa may be used with anticholinergic drugs, and this is useful when the tolerance limits of dosage have been reached. There is little advantage in using levodopa with amantadine, and when it is the unwanted effects are mainly attributable to the levodopa. Drugs are not satisfactory in the control of tremor, but may help sometimes.

Care is needed when the therapy is changed, as abrupt alterations in dosage may disturb the patient. If benzhexol is in use and levodopa is to be introduced, the benzhexol should be continued, or gradually reduced; if it is suddenly stopped, the patient may become rigid and think it is due to levodopa.

When a satisfactory dosage regime has been established, the patient should continue with it indefinitely. It is advisable for him to carry a card that records the current therapy.

Other Drugs in Parkinsonism. A further group of drugs that stimulate dopamine receptors, includes piribedil, apomorphine, and the ergot alkaloids bromocriptine and lergotrile. They all cause nausea, dyskinesia, and psychiatric disturbance to a degree that varies with the different drugs. Bromocriptine is the most promising. In addition to its dopaminergic effect, it suppresses pituitary function. The initial dose is 2·5 mg which may be increased slowly to 100 mg daily. The duration of action is 6 to 8 hours, and if combined with levodopa it is sometimes helpful in managing patients who show swings in response.

Surgical Treatment. Operations designed to relieve tremor have been in use for many years. The earlier methods such as cervical tractotomy reduced tremor by causing weakness of the affected muscles. Stereotactic methods made it possible to create a lesion deep in the cerebral hemisphere and to interrupt fibre pathways. A lesion in the lateral nucleus of the thalamus, for example, gives relief of tremor on the opposite side. Several methods are available, the lesion being caused by electrocoagulation or cryothermy.

There can be no doubt about the effect of a well-placed lesion in relieving or abolishing tremor, but there is no improvement in hypokinesia. The procedure became widespread during the decade before levodopa was introduced.

Unilateral thalamotomy carries a small risk of cerebral haemorrhage, hemiparesis, hemiballismus, and pulmonary embolism. Bilateral thalamotomy greatly increases the risk of complications and may be followed by disturbance of speech, equilibrium, and bulbar functions.

Stereotactic operations in Parkinsonism are now performed much less frequently. A unilateral operation may still be indicated when tremor is the main problem. If the tremor is unilateral it must be borne in mind that it may become generalised at a later stage. If the tremor is bilateral there may sometimes be a case for operation on one side. The patient may press for the other side to be done, but caution is needed because of the high incidence of complications.

Follow-up of patients submitted to operation has shown that success in the relief of tremor at an early stage may be followed by hypokinesia and other features as the disease progresses. It is therefore most important that a full medical assessment should be made before any operation is undertaken.

Supportive Therapy. Physiotherapy is of value in enabling the patient to adapt to increased activity when treatment is started, and of great importance after operation. A small proportion of patients remain severely incapacitated as a consequence of Parkinsonism. In the majority there is little place for long-term physiotherapy.

Parkinsonism and Hypertension. The association of systemic hypertension and Parkinsonism seems to be uncommon. When they coexist, the use of levodopa may relieve both disorders. Disturbing swings of blood pressure have been reported in patients under treatment with levodopa when given a general anaesthetic. Some normotensive patients become hypotensive when treated with levodopa, and a few of these complain of dizziness and a feeling of faintness that may be made worse by standing. These effects may be modified by reducing the dose or increasing it more gradually, but in a minority of the patients levodopa has to be stopped. The combination of levodopa and a monoamine oxidase inhibitor may cause hypertension and should be avoided.

In the *Shy-Drager syndrome* orthostatic hypotension is associated with features of Parkinsonism. It is commoner in males and usually develops between the ages of 50 and 70. The syndrome includes impotence, urinary and rectal incontinence, loss of sweating, iris atrophy, external ocular palsies, fasciculation and wasting of muscle, together with tremor, rigidity and loss of associated movements. Treatment is unsatisfactory. Fludrocortisone in a dosage of 0·1 to 0·6 mg daily may help to maintain blood pressure. Other measures are directed towards the reduction of pooling of blood in the lower limbs by applying pressure externally. Elastic stockings provide some support, but if a space suit is used a more effective pressure can be applied.

Steele-Richardson-Olszewski Syndrome (progressive supranuclear palsy). This disorder is characterised by mild features of Parkinsonism, mild dementia, a tendency to sudden falls, impairment of conjugate eye movements—particularly vertical gaze—and nuchal rigidity. Unfortunately, levodopa is relatively ineffective and only relieves the nuchal rigidity. There is no satisfactory treatment.

Parkinsonism and Dementia. Most patients with Parkinsonism show no gross signs of dementia. When dementia is prominent, both this and the extrapyramidal features may be attributable to encephalitis or other disease such as Jakob-Creutzfeld disease. The combination of Parkinsonism and dementia is also reported from certain closed communities such as the island of Guam where hereditary factors are probably important.

Drug-induced Parkinsonism. As already mentioned, the observation that reserpine might induce a Parkinsonian state led to important work on amines in the nervous system. Most of the drugs that produce this effect act by interfering with dopamine. Phenothiazines, tricyclic antidepressants, and butyrophenones block receptors. Reserpine and tetrabenazine modify storage.

Provided that the nature of the condition is recognised, it can be relieved by reducing the dose of the drug responsible. Anticholinergic drugs may also be of some value.

Wilson's disease is discussed in Chapter 20.

INVOLUNTARY MOVEMENTS

Tremor is defined as rhythmical involuntary movement of small amplitude. A physiological tremor at the rate of 10 Hz may be shown in normal adults and is brought out by movement. This physiological tremor is increased by anxiety, stress, and overaction of the thyroid gland. It is reduced by sedative drugs and beta blocking agents. Any tremor is likely to be made worse by anxiety and demonstration to an audience.

Benign Essential Tremor. Benign essential tremor is sometimes confused with Parkinsonism. The tremor usually affects the upper limbs, and the rate is 4 to 10 Hz. It continues through a movement, but is not accentuated and so differs from the intention tremor of cerebellar disorders. There may be a family history. Treatment is unsatisfactory. Small quantities of alcohol give relief and chlordiazepoxide 15 to 60 mg daily or diazepam 6 to 30 mg daily may help. Artane and beta blocking drugs are not generally effective but propranolol 40 mg t.d.s. may help, and the dose can be increased.

Tics. A tic is a repetitive involuntary movement of stereotyped form that commonly affects the face. Blepharospasm and sniffing are characteristic, but more complex movements also occur. In the child these movements are usually temporary. In the adult they may be provoked by stress, but when persistent they are difficult to treat. Drugs are not effective. Unravelling of any background psychopathology may help.

Hemifacial Spasm. This uncommon condition is of unknown aetiology and unilateral. It is usually seen in adults and consists of rhythmical contraction of the facial muscles often with closure of the eye. Facial weakness is usually present. Drug therapy is not effective. Reassurance and explanation may be sufficient. In persistent cases an injection of about 0·2 ml of 1 per cent phenol in glycerine into the facial nerve may give relief. The injection is usually made into a branch of the nerve distal to the parotid gland.

Chorea. Choreiform movement is seen in association with cerebral palsy in Sydenham's chorea and chorea gravidarum, as an effect of drugs such as levodopa, in Huntington's chorea, systemic lupus erythematosus, hyperthyroidism, polycythaemia rubra vera, and sometimes as an isolated feature in the elderly.

Huntington's chorea is occasionally seen in childhood, but usually develops in the third or fourth decade or later. It is characterised by choreiform movement, dementia, and deterioration in behaviour, with a family history. The mode of inheritance is autosomal dominant. Progression occurs, and in the later stages rigidity and other features of Parkinsonism may appear. The treatment of this distressing condition is unsatisfactory and there is no reliable means of predicting its development in an individual from an affected family. In such people small doses of levodopa may provoke involuntary movements, and this has been used in diagnosis.

Tetrabenazine (Nitoman) is useful in controlling choreiform movement, but the dose must be carefully adjusted. The initial dose is 25 mg daily by mouth. After a few days it may be increased to 25 mg twice daily, and later to 75 mg daily, but some patients are unable to tolerate the larger dose. Dosage is limited by drowsiness, depression, and hypokinetic effects. If this treatment fails, haloperidol 1·5 mg twice daily may be used and increased to 9 mg daily.

Hemiballismus resembles chorea, but the movements are unilateral and sometimes violent. The onset is usually sudden and vascular in aetiology. The condition may clear in a few weeks. Tetrabenazine may give relief. In persistent cases stereotactic thalamotomy on the side opposite to the movement is often effective.

Athetosis. Athetosis implies writhing involuntary movements which involve the limbs and may be associated with dystonia of the trunk. Athetosis occurs in patients with cerebral palsy, encephalitis, and Wilson's disease. It may follow hemiplegia or thalamotomy and is sometimes provoked by phenothiazines or butyrophenones. When treatment of the cause is not possible it is difficult to control the movements. Tetrabenazine, haloperidol, diazepam, and benzhexol are commonly used but are of limited value. Unilateral thalamotomy is sometimes helpful in patients with cerebral palsy.

Spasmodic Torticollis. The pathological basis of this is obscure. Much dispute has centred on the question of psychological factors. The established condition does not respond to psychiatric treatment. The presenting feature is a tendency to turn the head to one side, and there is commonly pain as well.

Treatment is difficult. Diazepam and benzhexol in large doses may control the movements. Tetrabenazine, haloperidol, and phenothiazines may sometimes give relief. Levodopa has been reported to help but has not relieved our patients. In severe cases the possibility of a stereotactic thalamotomy arises. It is only likely to be effective if done on both sides and can be combined with section of the accessory nerve and upper cervical motor roots on the side to which the head turns.

Torsion Dystonia. This uncommon condition may arise as a complication of anoxia, trauma at birth, or kernicterus but it is usually idiopathic. It may be sporadic or inherited as an autosomal dominant. Dystonic movements of the limbs, trunk, and neck occur. Progression is usual.

Treatment is unsatisfactory. In mild cases relief may be obtained by using the drugs mentioned under torticollis. Stereotactic thalamotomy may be performed in severe cases but the results are uncertain and there may be little relief. When the condition begins in childhood, disability is frequently severe. Onset in adult life may be associated with a benign course.

Writers Cramp. Mild forms are common and transient, but some patients develop tight contraction of the hand muscles combined with tremor and pain. The pressure exerted on the pen is often so great that it penetrates through the paper. The condition is similar to others that are linked with particular occupations such as violin playing or cigar making.

Writers cramp is occasionally a presenting feature of Parkinson's disease or associated with other neurological diseases, but in most cases it is an isolated feature. Treatment is difficult. Conditioning techniques that require the patient to trace out a pattern and give him a small electric shock when the pointer moves away from the pattern, have not proved successful in our hands. So far as writing is concerned, the best hope for the patient is to use the other hand. Behavioural psychotherapy may help, particularly with an obsessional patient. Supportive therapy with large doses of clomipramine may be useful.

Myoclonus (*see* page 73). Solitary myoclonic jerks are common in normal people and most often occur when at rest or falling asleep. Myoclonic jerks may also be seen in patients with epilepsy and, in the absence of other features of organic disease, they have a good prognosis. Myoclonus is associated with a variety of encephalopathies, some of which are familial and all of them are rare. Myoclonus is occasionally localised. It may then be attributable to spinal cord trauma, tumour, or inflammation.

The control of myoclonus is difficult. Some cases respond to anticonvulsant drugs. In a limited experience we have seen good results using clonazepam. The initial dose is 0·5 mg twice daily which is increased very gradually in steps of 0·5 mg. The limiting factor is drowsiness.

Recent reports indicate that L-5-hydroxytryptophane may reduce intention myoclonus (*see* page 12) and its potency is increased if it is combined with carbidopa. The oral daily dose of L-5 HT is in the range 100 to 1200 mg with carbidopa 25 to 200 mg. A full evaluation of this therapy is awaited. Tryptophane given alone would seem to have little effect.

9

Special Senses

Impairment of vision, auditory and vestibular function, smell and taste may be due to neurological disease but are frequently caused by disease of the sensory receptor.

Loss of vision is most commonly due to cataract, glaucoma, or disease of the retina, all of which can be diagnosed by examination of the eye. Deafness and vertigo may be due to disease of the peripheral vestibular and auditory apparatus. There is therefore a considerable overlap between specialties when dealing with disorders of the special senses.

OLFACTION AND TASTE

The distinction between anosmia and ageusia is important, and patients who complain of loss of taste are often found to have loss of smell sensation. Taste includes the recognition of salt, bitter, sweet and sour, and the appreciation of flavour depends on olfaction. Impairment of olfaction is more often due to disorder of the nose than of the olfactory nerve. The nerve may be contused or divided in a head injury, compressed by a tumour (meningioma) or granuloma, or involved in systemic disease. Some cases due to head injury recover in weeks or months. Anosmia may be due to psychological causes, and the hysterical patient may be unresponsive even to irritants such as ammonia. Testing should be done with familiar substances such as coffee, tar, and oil of cloves. Each nostril is tested separately and a useful distinction can be made between detection of the odour and identification of it. Bilateral loss of smell is a significant disability and deprives the patient of his appreciation of the flavour of food, scent of flowers, and other aromas. Persistent unilateral anosmia may indicate a compressive lesion of the olfactory nerve.

The anosmic patient is at some risk if exposed to coal gas, petrol, or exhaust fumes which he may not detect and which should be avoided.

Cerebrospinal rhinorrhoea may develop after head injury or cranial surgery and occurs in association with tumours. The patient is likely to develop meningitis and needs urgent investigation and treatment, usually by surgical closure of the leak.

Loss of taste may be due to disease involving the chorda tympani nerve. This is found in middle ear disease, and in some patients with a Bell's palsy. Ageusia is also present as a transient symptom after abdominal operations, as an unwanted effect of lithium and penicillamine, and in endocrine disorders, including hypothyroidism. Exceptionally it is sometimes found with anosmia after a head injury. The site of the lesion in this circumstance is unknown.

MANAGEMENT OF VISUAL FAILURE

The clinical history gives useful clues in seeking the cause of visual failure. Abrupt onset may favour a vascular basis while compression of a nerve is likely to cause progressive impairment. The physical examination must include measurement of the visual acuity, assessment of the visual fields, ophthalmoscopy, observation of the pupils and their responses, and consideration of the intraocular pressure. The patient may be unaware of a marked impairment of vision in one eye.

Visual acuity may be reduced because of refractive error, and for neurological purposes the corrected visual acuity is the significant finding. Poor vision due to refractive error may be improved by looking through a pinhole in a piece of paper. When the corrected visual acuity is subnormal it is important to establish the cause. If this is not apparent further investigation will be needed.

Loss of Vision in One Eye. The clinical history may indicate the probable pathology. Abrupt loss of vision in a previously healthy eye is likely to be due to vascular disease. In the older patient a history of headache, malaise, and, sometimes, joint pains will suggest cranial arteritis (page 56). A more gradual visual failure over several days with pain in the eye, in a young adult suggests optic neuritis. There may be a history of diplopia, paraesthesiae, or weakness, with remission which supports the diagnosis of multiple sclerosis. In acute glaucoma the eye is red and painful with oedema of the cornea and raised intraocular pressure. A gradual and progressive loss of vision over weeks or months suggests compression of the nerve and requires further investigation.

If the cornea, media and lens show no opacity, the retina is normal, and the intraocular pressure is satisfactory, the cause is likely to be related to the optic nerve. The optic disc may show swelling or pallor. The visual field usually shows a central scotoma which extends to the periphery at a later stage in cases of compression. The pupil reaction to light is lost if the eye is blind but in less severe cases the direct reaction on the side of the visual impairment is not well held (afferent pupillary sign).

The next step in investigation where compression is suspected is plain radiographs of the skull and optic foramina. There may be erosion of bone, enlargement of the optic foramina (suggesting optic nerve glioma—page 154), altered vascular markings, or an abnormal pituitary fossa. A meningioma of the sphenoidal ridge often causes bone erosion. If the plain radiographs are normal the possibility of craniopharyngioma, aneurysm, or meningioma may be pursued further. The computerised axial tomogram is of great value and may be supplemented by carotid arteriography or air encephalography. These modern radiological methods will usually demonstrate a compressive lesion and surgical treatment will then be required. If doubt remains and compression is suspected surgical exploration of the nerve is justified.

Many patients adapt quite quickly by using the healthy eye. Sometimes this is helped by temporary occlusion of the weak eye. A blind eye will tend to diverge as time passes.

Chiasmal Lesion. The clue here is the visual field defect which is classically a bitemporal hemianopia but often not typical. The visual loss is often asymmetrical. The optic disc may appear normal in the early stages of chiasmal compression. Erosion of the sella as seen in a lateral radiograph suggests a pituitary tumour (page 154). Plain radiographs may be normal in the presence of tumour or aneurysm. Further investigation may be required (Chapter 14).

Intrinsic disease of the chiasma due to vascular disorder, demyelinating disease, or glioma is relatively rare.

Postchiasmal Lesion. A unilateral lesion of the visual pathway behind the chiasma will produce a homonymous hemianopia. The commonest cause is vascular disease but a tumour may produce similar effects. The patient may be unaware of the visual disturbance and finds out about it when he collides with a doorpost, or with another vehicle when driving a car. A right homonymous hemianopia causes difficulty finding the beginning of a line of print. A left homonymous hemianopia leads to problems in reading successive lines. The use of a ruler placed across the page may relieve these difficulties.

The degree of adaptation that may occur after homonymous

hemianopia is remarkable and over a period of months the patient may overcome the disability although the field defect persists.

The loss of function after homonymous hemianopia is significantly greater than uniocular visual loss. The field of loss on the affected side is only partly compensated which makes driving a car hazardous.

Cortical and Subcortical Loss of Vision. Total visual loss may be due to bilateral disease of the occipital cortex or subcortical area. It is characteristic that the patient may be unaware of the visual defect, or even deny it. The pupil reactions and fundi are normal. The visual evoked response is absent.

Cortical visual loss of organic type must be distinguished from hysteria and this may cause difficulty when the signs of organic disease are scant. The patient with psychological disease tends to overact the part. He often bumps into objects deliberately and is inconsistent in performance. Observation when the patient is unaware may reveal activity that would not be possible without vision. When some vision is admitted there may be a gross discrepancy between subjective and objective findings. Patients with organic cortical visual loss can usually distinguish light from dark.

When the visual field is examined the patient with psychological disorder may show bizarre and rapidly fluctuating abnormalities. There may be gross constriction of the fields (tubular vision) but this also happens as a transient event in migraine, in the later phase of primary pigmentary degeneration of the retina, and with lesions of the occipital cortex that spare the occipital pole. A characteristic disturbance due to psychological disorder is the spiral field that constricts as it is plotted and then 'unwinds' when the direction of movement of the test object is reversed. Cortical blindness in an elderly patient of previously stable personality is unlikely to be due to psychological causes.

Visual loss due to vascular lesions may be transient but if it persists for more than a few hours it is likely to be permanent.

When visual loss is permanent suitable training may help the patient to deal with the disability. Results are best in the child or young adult. The use of a stick and guide dog may be taught as well as ordinary activities of daily living. Braille makes it possible for the patient to use written material. The radio and tape recorder help oral communication.

VERTIGO AND DEAFNESS

Vertigo is a subjective disturbance of orientation of the body in space.

The definition of the term implies a sense of rotation of the patient or surroundings, but a sense of falling or other forms of movement may be experienced. The sense of movement is within the head. Vertigo may be accompanied by pallor, sweating and vomiting. The patient is often extremely unsteady and past pointing and nystagmus may be demonstrated. The symptom may come on suddenly and with no particular reference to position or it may be induced by changes in posture.

Vague symptoms of dizziness may be due to feelings of depersonalisation seen in psychiatric disease. There is no sense of rotation but in many cases of psychogenic vertigo the patient feels tremulous and unsteady and constantly agitated. Light headedness and a swimming feeling in the head often precede syncope.

True vertigo has a wide variety of causes from peripheral ear disease and benign positional vertigo to more serious central causes such as multiple sclerosis, vertebrobasilar insufficiency, tumours in the region of the fourth ventricle, and temporal lobe epilepsy.

Most patients with deafness fall within the aegis of the otologist. The search for an acoustic neuroma in someone with progressive unilateral nerve deafness is important. Deafness is found in some hereditary disorders and may be associated with retinitis pigmentosa.

When vertigo and deafness occur together the lesion is usually in the peripheral part of the vestibular and auditory pathway.

Investigation. A complete history and examination will have revealed whether the deafness and vertigo are isolated or associated with other symptoms. The clinical examination must include an examination of the ear for old or active infection. The presence of a perforation of the drum precludes caloric testing in the affected ear.

Auditory Tests. Clinical tests of hearing may be misleading. The ability to hear whispered speech at a few feet or a ticking watch are the simplest tests. The tuning fork tests are helpful but sometimes unreliable. A fork vibrating at 256 and 512 Hz should be used. In Weber's test, a tuning fork placed centrally on the forehead may be referred to one or other ear. In conductive deafness referral is to the affected ear, in neural deafness to the unaffected ear. This is supplemented by Rinne's test when the tuning fork is placed adjacent to the external auditory meatus and over the mastoid process. Normally, air conduction is greater than bone conduction. In total deafness in one ear misleading results may be obtained due to spread of bone-conducted sound to the good ear. Refined audiometric testing is necessary to confirm the nature and severity of deafness. The results must be taken in conjunction with the clinical picture.

Pure tone audiometry compares air and bone conduction in five decibel steps at 128 to 8212 Hz in octaves. Masking of the opposite ear is necessary for bone conduction and for air conduction when hearing is impaired. This test indicates the presence of conductive or neural deafness or both.

Tests of loudness recruitment are useful in unilateral deafness. The ability of a deaf ear to hear loud sounds (100 decibels) just as well as a normal ear is characteristic of cochlear disorders but absent in nerve lesions and is of value in distinguishing a nerve lesion such as an acoustic neuroma from a cochlear lesion. Caution must be exercised in interpreting the test because a posterior fossa tumour may interfere with cochlear blood supply.

Speech discrimination is tested by masking one ear and asking the patient to repeat words without seeing the examiner's lips. The test can be quantified with a tape recording at 30 decibels above threshold using speech frequencies. A low score (few words heard), is suggestive of an auditory nerve lesion. Speech discrimination is impaired to a lesser extent in cochlear lesions.

Cortical evoked auditory potentials may be detected using computerised averaging techniques. In auditory nerve lesions the latency and amplitude are reduced. This is of value in young children and when non-organic disease is suspected in adults.

Vestibular Tests. The vestibular function tests are used to assess the side of the lesion and the level. Abnormalities of vestibular function are frequently bilateral.

A simple test utilises iced water (Linthicum). The head is tilted and 0·2 to 0·5 ml of iced water placed in the meatus. The water is allowed to stay in the ear for at least twenty seconds. The head is then displaced backwards 70°, and 30° forwards, and the subsequent nystagmus noted. A normal response is nystagmus in both positions for both ears.

The definitive procedure is the Fitzgerald-Hallpike test. Water at 30°C is run into the left ear for forty seconds and the nystagmus recorded from the time of starting irrigation. The same procedure is applied to the right ear. The procedure is repeated with water at 44°C. Cold water induces nystagmus away from the irrigated ear. Warm water produces nystagmus towards the irrigated ear. The nystagmus normally lasts about two minutes. A reduced duration of nystagmus in response to irrigating the same ear both with warm and cold water is termed canal paresis. Directional proponderance is the term applied when the hot and cold water nystagmus is induced in one direction to a much greater extent than the other; for example, directional proponderance to the right is when stimulation of the right ear with warm water and the left ear with cold water produces a much greater response than stimulation of the left ear with warm water and the right with cold water. Directional proponderance to the right can be due to a left lesion from the vestible to the inferior vestible nucleus or a right supratentorial lesion.

DEAFNESS IN CHILDHOOD

This problem usually involves the paediatrician, audiologist, otologist, and speech therapist rather than the neurologist. It may be very difficult to distinguish mental retardation, social deprivation and deafness. They may co-exist. Routine screening in school clinics has improved early diagnosis and remedial treatment with hearing aids, speech therapy, and attendance at a language school. Cortical evoked action potentials may be valuable in the diagnosis of deafness in early childhood.

ACOUSTIC NEUROMA

This is dealt with in Chapter 14. Progressive unilateral deafness without other signs is the stage at which the tumour should be diagnosed. Progressive unilateral neural deafness without loudness recruitment and poor speech discrimination suggest the diagnosis. Radiographs of the internal auditory meati may show unilateral erosion. A Myodil meatogram allows contrast media to enter the internal meatus and outline a small tumour. Computerised axial tomography may assist the diagnosis although its value in very small tumours has not been assessed.

MÉNIÈRE'S DISEASE

The triad of progressive neural deafness, tinnitus, and recurrent attacks of severe vertigo, constitute the clinical picture. The onset is often unilateral but may be bilateral. The pathological basis is an excess fluid content in the endolymphatic system. The cause is unknown. Familial examples occur.

The attacks of vertigo are violent and unpredictable. Fortunately, there may be a long remission between attacks. The vertigo may last for 24 hours or more and be associated with pallor, sweating, profuse vomiting and such a severe degree of rotary vertigo that the patient cannot move.

There is no cure for Ménière's disease. A wide variety of medicaments have been prescribed for the condition, including vasodilators, salt-free diet, and vitamins. The tinnitus and deafness have no specific treatment. Tinnitus may produce depression and a general lowering of morale. Sympathetic discussion of the problem together with the use of diazepam or an antidepressant may help. Diuretics, glycerol, and corticosteroids have all been tried but they are not established forms of treatment.

Medical treatment helps the nausea and vomiting and eases vertigo. However, the understanding of mechanisms underlying central vomiting and vertigo make rational therapy impossible and the extravagant claims for drugs cannot be justified.

Prochlorperazine maleate (Stemetil) 5 mg three times daily is widely used as a prophylactic for the vertigo and vomiting. In an acute attack 12·5 mg intramuscularly two or three times daily is helpful. Some drugs, notably betahistine hydrochloride (Serc) 8 mg three times daily, and cinnarizine (Stugeron) 15 to 30 mg three times daily are claimed to be of specific value in Ménière's disease and may help the cochlear symptoms. There is no evidence that these drugs are more effective than prochlorperazine. Other prophylactic drugs are prothipendyl hydrochloride (Tolnate) 10 mg three times daily and thiethylperazine maleate (Torecan) 10 mg t.d.s.

In the presence of intractable vertigo and vomiting a more radical approach is necessary. Although vertigo clears spontaneously at the end stage of the disease, operation may be required earlier. It may not be easy to decide which labyrinth is responsible for the vertigo. Caloric tests often indicate bilateral disease, often with a combination of canal paresis and directional proponderance.

The surgical treatment of Ménière's disease may be regarded as conservative, or destructive. Because the natural history is relatively benign only a small number of patients require radical surgery. A number of operations have been practised and one that has achieved considerable success is the endolymphatic subarachnoid shunt. Vertigo is improved in approximately 60 per cent of patients but the hearing response is variable. There is a risk of meningitis and haemorrhage. This operation has superseded simple incision of the saccus endolymphaticus. Drainage operations are suitable for patients with recurrent vertigo and there is an excellent chance of maintenance and occasional improvement in hearing.

Alternative procedures designed to preserve hearing are division of the intracranial portion of the vestibular nerve and ultrasonic destruction of the labyrinth. The operation on the vestibular nerve produces excellent results with regard to vertigo. The disadvantage is that it can only be performed in a small number of centres and has no influence on the natural history of the deafness. Ultrasonic operations on the vestibular end organ can control vertigo in up to 70 per cent of patients, and hearing deteriorates in about 25 per cent of operations. Tinnitus is often helped. The disadvantage of this operation is total deafness which may ensue in up to 5 per cent of cases.

Total destruction of the labyrinth should be avoided if possible. If the operation is carried out, a translabyrinthine approach is satisfactory. The destructive operation consists of removing the semicircular canals, utricle, saccule and endolymphatic duct. When tinnitus is a severe problem it is necessary to section the cochlear nerve.

In summary, the surgery of Ménière's disease varies from centre to centre. In the authors' view a drainage operation is the best initial procedure followed by ultrasonic treatment if required. The intracranial section of the vestibular nerve must be reserved for patients with little or no hearing loss and where facilities are available. Total destruction is rarely needed. Operations should be avoided in the elderly because many old people become very unsteady.

VESTIBULAR NEURONITIS

The disorder is self limiting and of obscure origin. It may be sporadic or appear in epidemics associated with a viral infection. The site of the lesion is unknown. The caloric tests are bilaterally abnormal. Attacks of severe vertigo may persist for several weeks but then usually cease. Occasionally there is a relapse. The non-recurring nature of the symptoms, the absence of auditory symptoms and the association with viral infection distinguish it from Ménière's disease. Parenteral prochlorperazine is beneficial in the stage of acute vertigo. Reassurance about the benign self-limiting course of the disease is important.

POSITIONAL VERTIGO

Positional vertigo may be due to peripheral or central lesions. The term benign positional vertigo should be avoided as it implies that it is easily distinguished from other more significant varieties.

In one type of positional vertigo the sensation fatigues on repeated manoeuvring the head into the precipitating position. In other cases it persists unchanged.

The view that the first type indicated disease of the utricle and that persistent positional vertigo was due to central disease is an oversimplification and misleading.

For the purposes of clinical examination, vertigo may be induced by lowering the patient's head over the couch 30 degrees below the horizontal with the head turned to one side and one ear upwards. After a short lag, nystagmus is induced with the fast component downwards towards the lowermost ear. Repeating the manoeuvre may fatigue the response or it may persist unchanged.

A careful search should be made for central nervous system disease in all patients with positional vertigo. Many examples are benign and resolve spontaneously. This is particularly so in the young. Positional vertigo following head injury may persist for up to two years. The triad of headache, vomiting, and positional vertigo may indicate a tumour in the fourth ventricle.

When a structural disease such as multiple sclerosis or a posterior fossa tumour is found, treatment is directed to the basic disease process.

OTHER CAUSES OF VERTIGO

Migraine may be associated with vertigo in the acute attack. Vertigo in migraine represents involvement of the posterior circulation or the temporal lobes.

Transient ischaemic attacks in the vertebrobasilar territory may cause vertigo in isolation, or with other symptoms. If hypertension is present, adequate control of the blood pressure may relieve the symptoms. In normotensive extracranial vascular disease anticoagulants may be used. The use of aspirin and sulphinpyrazone 200 mg t.d.s., to reduce platelet adhesiveness are under trial. The role of surgery in extracranial vascular disease is discussed in Chapter 12. Vertigo is a prominent symptom in the lateral medullary syndrome. Sudden vertigo with or without deafness and with recovery often taking place over several weeks may be due to occlusion of the internal auditory artery.

Multiple sclerosis may cause recurrent attacks of vertigo. Other symptoms and signs usually suggest the disease. Apart from symptomatic treatment corticosteroid therapy may be indicated if the vertigo is part of an acute relapse (page 115). Recurrent brief attacks of vertigo in multiple sclerosis occasionally respond to carbamazepine.

A neoplasm in the brain stem and, in particular, in the region of the fourth ventricle, may cause recurrent vertigo. Early diagnosis can only be made by neuroradiological studies which would now include computerised transverse axial tomography. At a later stage there is raised intracranial pressure.

Temporal lobe epilepsy has many manifestations and a brief aura of vertigo may herald an attack. The vertigo is not isolated and is accompanied by other evidence of temporal lobe dysfunction. The treatment is as for other forms of temporal lobe epilepsy.

Streptomycin and related antibiotics cause vestibular damage, which is permanent. Compensation may take place in the young. Unfortunately, the complication is commoner in the elderly and those with poor renal function. Awareness of the possibility is the most important aspect of drug-induced vertigo.

10

Dementia and Degenerative Disorders

Dementia refers to an acquired intellectual deterioration that may involve changes in mood and behaviour and is frequently progressive. A non-progressive situation may follow head injury or infection. Dementia due to diffuse organic brain disease must be differentiated from pseudodementia due to functional psychiatric illness and focal cerebral lesions. Mental subnormality refers to a failure of development of normal higher mental activity. This chapter deals with the assessment and management of dementia in adults. In addition, the management of a number of degenerative disorders, some of which are associated with dementia, are dicussed.

ASSESSMENT OF DEMENTIA

Clinical History. The patient, relatives, and friends may all give relevant information on the time scale and pattern of altered behaviour. The patient's inability to cope with a job, poor memory, mental confusion, difficulty in finding his way around, and altered mood and personality may all be present. In taking the clinical history, it is important to decide whether the symptomatology may be explained on the basis of a focal lesion such as a brain tumour, or whether the apparent symptoms of dementia could be due to an affective disorder such as endogenous depression. The pattern of the history and the appearance of the patient often make the basic diagnosis of dementia easy. However, in the history, one must note whether there is any specific disorder such as dysphasia which might suggest a focal lesion. Other aspects of the history such as drug and alcohol intake, the presence of symptoms suggestive of systemic disease, or the addition of other neurological symptoms such as headache or motor disability must be sought.

Examination. The examination should include a full appraisal of mental function. Orientation in time and place should be the first facts assessed, followed by the name and address. Other aspects of mental performance are affected by this information. The patient's mood is noted. Questions of simple general knowledge such as the name of the Prime Minister, the Queen's children or local facts of universal interest are asked. The presence of dysphasia may already have been noted. Minor degrees of language difficulty can be shown by asking the patient to put the right word to a verbal description of a periscope, stethescope and telescope. These questions eliminate tactile and visual clues. They can be modified according to intelligence. Naming five or ten types of flower may bring out language problems.

The ability to retain numerals can be tested with digit retention. A normal person should be able to retain six digits forwards. Verbal learning is often tested by the Babcock sentence which, in normal people, may be repeated correctly at the first or second attempt. The inability to register and recall simple facts over one to three minutes tests recent memory. Adding and subtraction and a serial sevens test assess calculation.

Assessment on performance in tests of mental function must be made on the basis of the patient's total performance. Clouding of consciousness and disorientation will make specific statements impossible. The use of tests such as Koh's blocks for constructional apraxia are of value only if information about colour vision, the visual fields, and specific motor and sensory defects is known. Nevertheless, clinical tests of mental function are valuable and if applied with patience yield information that may be just as valuable as formal psychometry.

The mental testing must be associated with a full neurological examination and a systems review. This need not necessarily be carried out at the same session. There is much to be said for carrying out a minimal assessment of mental function to assist in the remainder of the physical examination, and then to return to mental testing over several individual sessons.

Differential Diagnosis. Dementia must be distinguished from endogenous depression or schizophrenia. A flat affect, motor retardation, and general mental sluggishness may lead to misdiagnosis of a functional psychosis as dementia. The presence of delusions and hallucinations in a clear consciousness and other features of schizophrenia may assist in this diagnosis but it is quite common to confuse depression and dementia in the elderly. A response to a therapeutic trial of antidepressants is sometimes the best way to resolve doubt. It is necessary to remember that the presence of cerebral atrophy in the elderly does not exclude a diagnosis of depression.

Involuntary movements such as chorea or myoclonus raise the possibilities of Huntington's chorea or the Jakob-Creutzfeldt syndrome. Pyramidal signs, ataxia, and incontinence make the diagnosis of normal pressure hydrocephalus a possibility. A variety of physical signs as well as pupillary changes raise the possibility of neurosyphilis. There may also be pointers to vitamin B12 deficiency or hypothyroidism.

Investigations. A chest X-ray may indicate pulmonary lesions suggestive of primary or secondary carcinoma. Skull radiographs occasionally show an unsuspected area of calcification or a shifted pineal. The EEG may show abnormalities suggestive of a focal or diffuse disturbance. Specific tests may indicate pernicious anaemia, hypothyroidism, syphilis, or chronic renal and hepatic disease. A brain scan may indicate a focal lesion. Computerised axial transverse tomography of the brain will show ventricular size and the degree of cortical atrophy. Invasive techniques such as air encephalography will show similar findings but with more distress to the patient, including headache and sometimes increased mental confusion. Brain biopsy may be indicated but in many instances the procedure produces inconclusive results. It should be undertaken only when there is a specific diagnosis in mind.

Psychometry. In gross cases of dementia, psychometry is of little value and cannot be applied with any accuracy. The true value of psychological testing is a matter for dispute in progressive dementia. It will help to distinguish between diffuse cerebral involvement and a focal process. It may indicate the presence or absence of dementia when there is doubt whether the condition is organic or functional. The Wechsler adult intelligence scale is reliable and reproducible. It consists of a number of tests covering verbal and performance abilities which are scored and from which a verbal and performance intelligence quotient can be calculated. It may be corrected for age. Normally, the performance scale falls off in relation to the verbal scale, except when there is dysphasia. A deterioration quotient can be calculated and certain aspects of performance such as vocabulary tend to be preserved and given an indication of previous intelligence. In dementia following head injury, psychometry may be used to follow progress and guide rehabilitation. In mental subnormality, psychometry gives an indication of overall function and delineates more specific defects. It may show up the child who is in fact intelligent, apart from developmental dyslexia, and who has been labelled as subnormal.

MANAGEMENT OF SPECIFIC DISORDERS

The object of investigating all patients with dementia is to exclude a treatable cause. Unfortunately, it is relatively rare to find a treatable disease. Notable exceptions are the metabolic dementias due to vitamin B12 deficiency and hypothyroidism. The diagnosis of neurosyphilis may result in a good response to penicillin treatment, and some patients regarded as having a diffuse degenerative disorder have benign removable brain tumours. Occasionally, the relatively acute onset of dementia without physical signs may be caused by a subdural haematoma.

Provided treatable disease is excluded, the general outline of management is common to most causes. Malnutrition due to self neglect should be corrected. An assessment must be made of the patient's ability to cope on his own or with some help in the community. Such an assessment can be made by an occupational therapist and social worker in conjunction with the hospital doctor and general practitioner. Most patients with moderate dementia will need family support at the least. They will be unable to shop, manage the house or keep themselves out of danger. If the patient is very restless great problems may ensue; for instance, a retired bank manager made telephone calls and tried to attend non-existent meetings at all times of the day and night! Patients may be prone to antisocial behaviour and urinate in inappropriate places, expose themselves, or make uninhibited remarks. If the patient becomes unmanageable, then long-term care in a mental hospital is required. This may be needed at an early stage if there is little community support. Unfortunately, western civilisation is much less effective in this respect than many civilisations in the third world.

Alzheimer's and Pick's Disease. These conditions develop insidiously in middle age or later, and they are occasionally found in younger age groups. Pick's disease is a more focal disorder and may be inherited as an autosomal dominant. Alzheimer's disease is normally sporadic. Both conditions progress insidiously and long-term care is often required. It is distressing to observe the deterioration in mental function, and difficult to know how much the patient suffers. There are frequently moments of anguish and brief insight.

Many elderly patients have Alzheimer's disease and not arteriosclerotic dementia. The identity of arteriosclerotic dementia is a controversial matter. Patients with a history of multiple infarcts may develop dementia but there is usually a clear-cut history of previous stroke episodes. In the case of multiple lacuna infarcts associated with hypertension, the history may be less convincing. There is no treatment for dementia due to Alzheimer's or Pick's disease. Despite this, brain biopsy is sometimes recommended. It is seldom justified, and the information may be non-specific. Biopsy may be followed by the development of epilepsy. There is no evidence that vasodilator drugs, some of which are said to have a more direct effect on metabolism, are of any value. Shunt operations using a low pressure value have been tried but they are ineffective.

Huntington's Chorea. The choreiform movements associated with this disorder are covered in Chapter 8. There is a rigid form that is occasionally found in childhood and early adult life. In any family in which Huntington's chorea exists, it is important to examine all members who may develop the disease. Since the condition is an autosomal dominant each child of an affected parent has a 50 per cent chance of inheriting the disease. Early signs may be mild changes in behaviour and affect. The restlessness due to minor choreiform movements is easily missed without careful observation. If the diagnosis can be made before reproduction has taken place appropriate genetic advice may be given. In practice this seldom happens. The levodopa test was designed in an attempt to produce choreiform movements in a much smaller dose than would normally be the case. The test is unreliable and there is anxiety about precipitating the clinical features prematurely.

Dementia or involuntary movements may predominate. Sometimes the patient presents with behavioural abnormalities, even with a sexual offence. There is some help for the involuntary movements by using tetrabenazene 25 to 225 mg daily. The higher dose may made the patient drowsy and depressed and cause nausea, anorexia and vomiting. Thiopropazate (Dartalan) 5 to 10 mg t.d.s. is an alternative.

Neurosyphilis. This is now a rare cause of dementia and is dealt with in Chapter 19.

VIRUS INFECTIONS

A number of specific virus infections may be associated with dementia. In most instances the dementia is non-progressive but in subacute sclerosing panencephalitis the disease runs a relapsing progressive course.

The dementia associated with herpes simplex encephalitis is dealt with in Chapter 19. Unfortunately, the mortality and morbidity with this illness is high. The temporal lobes are selectively damaged and survivors may exhibit gross memory disturbance, a voracious appetite, and hypersexuality. Permanent care may be needed.

Encephalitic illness associated with arthropod-borne viruses are rare in the UK but can cause dementia. Encephalitic illness related to a variety of infections and exanthemata may cause serious brain damage due to demyelination. A similar picture may follow rabies and smallpox vaccination. Steroids are used for these conditions but the real value of this medication is unproven.

Subacute sclerosing panencephalitis is due to measles infection with an altered immune response. As a rule it is found in children and the course is relapsing and usually fatal. Partial recovery and arrest of the condition is recorded. The treatment for this condition has been varied. Amantadine, corticosteroids, thymectomy, and transfer factor have all been tried. There is no definite evidence that any of these is effective.

The myoclonic jerks in this condition may be helped by clonazepam, or sodium valproate. The child can be managed at home with suitable support until the terminal phase.

Normal Pressure Hydrocephalus. This condition presents with dementia, incontinence, and pyramidal and cerebellar signs. The ventricular system is grossly enlarged. Air encephalography is poorly tolerated and there is a failure of air to flow over the cerebral hemisphere. A radio-iodinated serum albumin scan (RISA scan) shows delayed clearance of isotope from the ventricles after it has been injected into the lumbar theca. Computerised axial tomography is a simpler and safer way of demonstrating ventricular size and cortical atrophy but it has not been shown to be a more reliable diagnostic technique.

Difficulty has arisen in identifying this condition. Appearances on air encephalography and scanning are not diagnostic. The treatment of normal pressure hydrocephalus is to insert a low pressure valve shunt. The results have been disappointing in many instances probably because of poor case selection and a long-standing history. There are good operative results in some patients, particularly when there is evidence of a precipitating factor such as meningitis or subarachnoid haemorrhage.

Metabolic Dementia. There are a number of causes of metabolic dementia, some of which are treatable.

In hypothyroidism the patient may become slow, apathetic and confused and even be misdiagnosed as having endogenous depression. The striking 'myxoedema madness' described by Richard Asher is a florid psychosis in which the patient is noisy, quarrelsome, and even violent. Hypothyroid dementia responds in most cases to thyroxine provided the diagnosis is made at an early stage.

Hypoadrenalism may produce a psychosis and mental confusion but other symptoms usually predominate. Hyperadrenalism in Cushing's syndrome can cause a psychosis and a similar situation may develop in response to steroid therapy or a hormone-producing carcinoma of the bronchus.

The effects of hypoglycaemia, disturbances of calcium metabolism and hepatic and renal disease are discussed in Chapter 20.

One form of dementia of unknown aetiology related to renal disease is *dialysis dementia.* This may be the cause of death in some patients on chronic haemodialysis. It usually occurs after fifteen to eighteen months' treatment, but may appear after several years. Speech disturbance, myoclonus, akinetic mutism and a global dementia develop. The patient may become agitated, paranoid and develop focal motor signs. Investigations are unhelpful although the EEG shows an excess of high voltage slow waves. All treatment has been ineffective. This includes increased dialysis frequency, renal transplantation, levodopa, and penicillamine. It has been suggested that the encephalopathy may be due to intoxication with trace elements, possibly aluminium.

Dementia Associated with Malignant Disease. Progressive dementia may develop as a non-metastatic complication of malignancy or be due to metastases. In the latter there may be extensive physical signs, and multiple lesions on a brain scan or computerised tomogram.

A chronic form of limbic encephalitis has been reported in association with carcinoma, mainly involving the temporal lobes. It may be combined with other non-metastatic neurological complications. There is no effective treatment.

Multifocal leucoencephalopathy is a demyelinating disorder associated with malignancy. Multifocal demyelination occurs with varying physical signs, often presenting with an organic psychosis and rapidly evolving to severe dementia. A polyoma virus has been implicated. Corticosteroids and immunosuppressants have been tried without effect.

Slow Virus Infections. The Jakob-Creutzfeldt syndrome is a rapid form of dementia developing over months, associated with a variety of additional signs including myoclonus, cortical blindness, extrapyramidal and pyramidal signs and involvement of the lower motor neurone. The disease is transmissible to chimpanzees and spider monkeys. The EEG shows reduction of normal activity with frequent generalised sharp wave complexes. There is no effective treatment. Corticosteroids and antiviral agents have been tried without success. The patient is likely to need continuous hospital care. Skilled nursing helps but the quality of life is poor.

Kuru is a localised transmissible disease found in a highland tribe in New Guinea who ingested infected human brains. The disease produces cerebellar signs and dementia. It is possible to abolish the condition by stopping cannibalism. The disease is now dying out.

Leucodystrophies and Storage Diseases. These conditions form a large group of metabolic disorders most often inherited as an autosomal recessive. They are usually childhood disorders, although an adult form of metachromatic leucodystrophy is described. It is beyond the scope of this book to describe these conditions in detail. Research is directed towards finding the basic enzyme deficiency and achieving antenatal diagnosis by amniocentesis and measurement of the enzyme in the amniotic cell. The same principle is applied to enzyme measurement in white blood cells in suspected patients.

One of the commoner examples is metachromatic leucodystrophy inherited as an autosomal recessive and due to deficiency of the enzyme aryl sulphatase. The enzyme deficiency may be measured in urine, washed leucocytes, or skin fibroblasts. The condition may be diagnosed by amniocentesis in suspected cases. The onset may be in early life, childhood, or adult life. The progression is slower in the later onset cases. There is a combination of pyramidal tract, peripheral nerve, and cerebellar involvement. Dementia is a universal feature. Slowing of peripheral nerve conduction is a helpful diagnostic feature when the disease is suspected.

Unfortunately, none of these conditions is treatable and all that can be offered is general support and genetic advice to the parents which is facilitated when the disease can be diagnosed in utero.

DEGENERATIVE DISORDERS

Some system degenerative disorders may be associated with dementia but many are not. The cerebellar and spinocerebellar degenerations are only occasionally associated with severe dementia. They are dealt with in this chapter because they are chronic progressive diseases of unknown cause and in this respect have much in common with presenile dementia.

Multisystem Degeneration (Shy-Drager Syndrome). This disorder occurs in middle age or later and is characterised by severe postural hypotension, pyramidal cerebellar and extrapyramidal features and urinary incontinence. Severe dementia may sometimes be evident but it is rare. Other evidence of autonomic system involvement is failure to sweat and an abnormal valsalva manoeuvre. The neurological features are untreatable but postural hypotension may be treated by fludrocortisone 0·1 to 0·6 mg daily. In extreme circumstances an antigravity suit may be used. There may be postural hypotension without other neurological features.

Cerebellar Degenerations. Olivo-ponto-cerebellar degeneration is rare and may be sporadic or inherited as a dominant trait. Pyramidal and extrapyramidal signs exist and in some patients there is dementia. Sometimes rigidity can be helped by drugs such as benzhexol but there is no specific treatment. The olivo-cerebellar type described by Holmes is inherited as a dominant. There is no treatment. The subacute cerebellar degeneration associated with carcinoma does not respond to treatment. The theoretical possibility that the condition might be improved if the carcinoma is eradicated never seems to apply.

Ataxia telangiectasia is a rare disorder presenting in childhood. The neurological manifestations include severe cerebellar ataxia and athetoid movements. Telangiectasia are seen around the eye. There is an associated immunoglobulin deficiency predisposing to repeated infections. The disease is progressive and most patients die at an early age. The administration of repeated courses of antibiotics is necessary to combat infection.

Friedreich's Ataxia. This condition may have a dominant or recessive inheritance. It is associated with pes cavus, scoliosis, ataxia, absent reflexes, particularly in the lower limb, and extensor plantar responses. There is position sense loss in the toes.

There may be heart disease and diabetes mellitus. Optic atrophy, deafness and retinitis pigmentosa may also be present. Cardiomyopathy may be the cause of sudden death. Heart failure is common and needs treatment with digoxin and diuretics. There is no specific therapy. Care must be taken to try to prevent the scoliosis from progressing to severe deformity. Operations to overcome tightening of the tendo achillis will improve the position of the foot and the problem of footwear. Many of these patients live a wheelchair existence by their early twenties.

11

Multiple Sclerosis

Multiple sclerosis (MS) is the commonest of the demyelinating diseases of the central nervous system. Devic's disease (neuromyelitis optica) is closely related and regarded by many as a variant of MS in which the disease process attacks the optic nerves and spinal cord. Schilder's disease is rare and begins as a subcortical disorder. The other types of encephalomyelitis are discussed in Chapter 19.

Subacute myelo-optic neuropathy (SMON) was common in Japan and seemed to be induced by taking large doses of clioquinol (Entero-Vioform). The pathological finding was demyelination of tracts in the central nervous system.

The first clinical manifestation of MS usually appears between puberty and the age of 50 and it is twice as common in women as in men. The course and severity show marked variation. We know little of the aetiology. It may be acquired in childhood but is seldom manifest before the age of 17 years. Only about 3 per cent of the patients have a close relative with the disease. Virus infection, altered immunity, and diet may contribute. The IgG component of spinal fluid is increased. The histocompatibility antigens HLA A2, HLA B7 and HLA Dw2 are often increased. Antibodies to basic myelin protein have not been demonstrated. The brain shows a reduced content of unsaturated fatty acids. Trauma, infection, and pregnancy may provoke an exacerbation of the disease.

Diagnosis. The diagnosis of MS is difficult in the early stages. Often it is suspected when the evidence is insufficient to make it more than a possibility. There is no specific laboratory test but examination of the spinal fluid may help. An increase in lymphocytes up to 60/mm^3 may occur in the acute exacerbation but the most constant feature is an increase in gammaglobulin above 0·05 g/litre. The total protein may be slightly increased but rarely exceeds 1·0g/litre (normal 0·20 to 0·40 g/litre).

The problem of early diagnosis leads to difficulties in communication between doctor and patient and sometimes between doctors. A firm diagnosis is to be avoided where doubt exists, but patients are increasingly aware of the disease and more often ask direct questions. In such circumstances it is reasonable to speak of inflammation of the nerve centres to the patient and in medical terms of a possible episode of demyelination. From this it should not be assumed that progression to MS is inevitable. Some isolated features such as optic neuritis do not show inevitable progression to the generalised disease. But some patients will not accept these explanations which, in turn, may provoke various attitudes on the part of the doctor. He may be evasive and is then accused of 'not telling me anything'. The doctor may tell the patient that he has MS when the diagnosis is doubtful and this, in turn, may be received in various ways. The patient may reject the diagnosis and seek other opinions, perhaps followed by investigations to exclude other disorders; or may accept the diagnosis and reject the doctor, concluding that there is no specific therapy and that as the course is unpredictable medical supervision has little to offer. There can be no doubt about the difficulty of handling the patient with persistent symptoms for which no definite cause can be stated and no effective treatment provided. Fortunately, the position is not one of unrelieved gloom, because spontaneous remission of symptoms and signs is often a feature in the early stages of the disease.

MANAGEMENT

Management will be considered under the headings—

1 Early stage
2 Established disease.

1 EARLY STAGE

The presenting feature is commonly unilateral visual loss, double vision, paraesthesiae, weakness or numbness of one or more limbs, vertigo, or ataxia. The clinical picture may suggest a spinal cord lesion, and certainly myelopathy may be an early feature of the disease but special caution is needed if the signs are confined to this area. A myelogram will nearly always be required to exclude a compressive lesion. Examination of the patient will often reveal physical signs indicating more widespread disease than the symptoms suggest. Paucity of signs or neglect of the physical examination may lead to the diagnosis of hysteria, and sometimes it is exceedingly difficult to be sure about the organic nature of the symptoms. Where such doubt exists it is usually wise to await events. While resolution of the symptoms or signs will please the patient it is a valuable point in making the diagnosis. The occurrence of a remission is easily but wrongly attributed to the current drug therapy.

If an episode of demyelination is suspected what should be done? Many authors advise rest in bed, which becomes inevitable if there is marked weakness, vertigo, or gross ataxia. When the features are less severe the value of bed rest is debatable, and some authorities have actually recommended exercise. Reduced activity is usually wise. In practical terms it is impossible for a housewife to rest at home. This raises the question whether admission to hospital is to be advised. It may be the best course if the symptoms are severe because it provides an opportunity for lumbar puncture and other investigations, and it convinces the patient that the symptoms are being taken seriously. On the other hand, a young woman with acute optic neuritis or diplopia may gain little from admission to hospital. Hospital admission may actually lead to new problems. The patient admitted to a neurological unit will almost certainly meet a patient with advanced MS and it may well be that his or her disease began in the same way. Such a revelation gives little comfort.

It is at this early stage of disease that effective treatment might produce its greatest benefit. At present no such therapy is available and the diagnosis of MS is less urgent. It is important that new therapies should be properly evaluated in special units where experience of the disease and an adequate number of patients is available. Remission is common. The most valuable criterion for assessment of a new drug is its capacity to prevent relapse.

General Measures. Adequate nutrition, control of obesity, and moderation of habits are obviously desirable. Vitamin therapy has often been used but there is no evidence that it alters the natural course of the disease. As a harmless placebo the vitamin B complex or injections of hydroxycobalamin may have a place in treatment.

It seems clear that infection may aggravate the disease temporarily, and general measures should be combined with specific antibiotic or chemotherapy when there is a firm indication.

Pregnancy. If the patient is pregnant for the first time the effect on the disease is unpredictable. On general grounds it is better to avoid pregnancy during the active phase of the disease. When it does arise, the question of termination of the pregnancy may be raised. This requires a review of the patient's physical condition, disability, age, number of children, religious views and attitudes. It must also take account of the prognosis and the difficulties presented to a mother in looking after a young child.

Relapse sometimes occurs during the puerperium. There is no clear evidence that the contraceptive pill aggravates the disease. When the disability is severe, sterilisation may be the best course and is usually advised when a pregnancy is terminated.

Table 11.1 Treatment Regimes in Multiple Sclerosis

A Acute exacerbation

1 Dexamethasone 2 mg three times daily for 5 days.

2 Prednisolone 40 to 80 mg daily or corticotrophin 40 units by IM injection for a month followed by gradual withdrawal over the next fortnight.

3 (only in hospital with full facilities)
Methyl prednisolone 1 g intravenously daily for 7 days followed by prednisolone 30 mg daily for a week and gradual withdrawal over the next fortnight.

B Chronic disease

1 Gluten-free diet.

2 Avoidance of saturated fats in the diet combined with sunflower oil 30 to 60 ml daily.

Steroid Therapy. Corticosteroid therapy, ACTH, or tetracocactrin (Synacthen) have been recommended as treatment in the acute exacerbation. This treatment may shorten the duration of an exacerbation and it probably acts by controlling the associated oedema of the brain and spinal cord. There is no evidence that it modifies the course of the disease and it does *not* prevent relapse. Claims that ACTH is more effective than corticosteroid may be explained by relative dosage equivalents. A suitable course of treatment would be corticotrophin, tetracosactrin 1 mg on alternate days by intramuscular injection for a month, or prednisolone by mouth. Each course would last for about one month (Table 11.1).

The usual contra-indications to this therapy should be remembered and it is better avoided in the presence of peptic ulcer, infection, psychosis, or thrombosis of a limb vein. It is justified in a severe acute exacerbation. If it is continued for longer than a month other untoward effects become prominent, and moreover, the treatment is without effect in the inactive phase of the disease. Unfortunately, patients are inclined to attribute an early remission to this therapy and become conditioned to expect a similar response in later episodes which may not occur. (*See also* Chapter 20.)

Alternative Drug Therapy. It is inevitable that in a chronic disease for which there is no specific treatment various remedies should gain favour. They range from potent and toxic drugs to harmless placebos. Azathioprine is a cytotoxic drug that suppresses immune mechanisms. A controlled trial over a period of two years has shown that a dose of 200 mg daily will not prevent relapses (Swinburn and Liversedge, 1973). Combinations of vitamins and antibiotics are sometimes advised but ineffective except in so far as they control secondary infection. The Russian vaccine, a modified rabies vaccine which became a popular therapy, is not merely ineffective, but potentially harmful. Antilymphocytic serum is currently under trial. There are favourable reports of the use of transfer factor. More drastic measures include total immunosuppression combined with corticosteroids in high doses and antilymphocytic globulin but this is not an established form of therapy.

Diet. Current attitudes favour a dietary approach. This derives from the appreciation that loss of specific lipid constituents of myelin is an early feature of the disease and the inference that lipid metabolism is disordered.

The gluten-free diet has been found effective in coeliac disease and some cases of adult steatorrhoea, but there is no evidence of gluten intolerance in MS. The diet requires the use of special flour for bread, cakes, pastry, and similar foods. The flour is more expensive than the usual variety and the food products are only available in the larger towns. Presumably the treatment could be effective only in the long term, and its value is not established. Trials are continuing. It can be said that the diet does not seem to be harmful although some patients lose weight. Some patients have developed exacerbations of disease while keeping to this diet.

Claims are also made for the addition of unsaturated fatty acids, notably linoleic acid, to the diet. This can be given in the form of sunflower seed oil in the dose 30 to 60 ml daily. The oil is unpalatable and many patients do not tolerate the larger dose. Linoleic acid is available in tablet form.

Physiotherapy. In the acute stage this should be directed to passive movement of the limbs and prevention of contracture and deformity. Later, it can be more active, and graduated exercises help to ensure maximum function and aid postural mechanisms. Little is gained by regular attendance over long periods. It is better to use short courses of treatment for guidance and encouragement at critical points in the course of the disease. Physiotherapy may prove to be too exhausting for the severely disabled.

Vaccination and Immunisation. The injection of preparations containing animal protein is better avoided when possible and vaccines may provoke an exacerbation of disease. In the course of an epidemic the relative risks of using or avoiding this procedure must be weighed.

Hospital Supervision. Whether the patient should attend the hospital for follow-up can be considered at this point. Much will depend on the liaison established between patient, general practitioner, and consultant. If there has been a remission and disability is minimal or absent there is often little purpose in routine attendance at the hospital. Where some symptoms persist, or fluctuate, regular follow-up can provide support and ensure that help is provided when it is needed. At this stage the patient is often the recipient of inconsiderate remarks such as accusations of drunkenness when walking or advice to 'get something done about it'. Supervision by the general practitioner or hospital provides a buffer in this situation and avoids multiple medical consultations when new symptoms arise or old problems persist. This type of supervision is much more satisfactory when the patient is seen by the same doctor at each visit.

2. THE ESTABLISHED DISEASE

At this stage the diagnosis is no longer in reasonable doubt and there are some persistent symptoms or signs. The various clinical features will be discussed in relation to management. It is often found that exercise, or a rise in body temperature such as may result from a hot bath, will aggravate the symptoms temporarily.

Visual Symptoms. Acute optic neuritis (retrobulbar neuritis) is associated with pain, tenderness of the globe, visual failure and central scotoma. In most cases the pain settles in about a week and vision recovers in about six weeks. While most cases make a substantial recovery, about a sixth have persistent visual disturbance. There are some patients in whom involvement of the optic nerves is insidious and progressive without an acute episode of visual failure. Prognosis for recovery of vision is generally good in the acute episode, but less favourable in those with insidious visual failure. Occasionally, the visual loss is severe and permanent.

In those with severe visual loss, telescopic devices may allow the patient to read but may be difficult to use if there is associated tremor or ataxia. Registration as blind or partially sighted may facilitate social benefits such as a radio, payment for some necessities, and, where appropriate, a guide dog.

Diplopia occurs in disease of the brain stem. Sometimes it is associated with ophthalmoplegia or an ocular muscle palsy but often the palsy is minimal. A few patients are slow to find out that relief can be obtained by covering one eye. Some patients are helped by reassurance that no harm will be done by using the eyes or occluding one of them.

Trigeminal Neuralgia and Neuropathy. This is uncommon but is found in those with brain-stem disease. The neuralgia may be exactly similar to that seen in the elderly who have no gross disease. The pain is unilateral and, usually, in the second or third division of the trigeminal nerve distribution. It is brief, excruciating, and recurrent. It is provoked by contact with the face and by washing, eating, or exposure to a cold wind. Usually, there is some sensory loss over the face.

Carbamazepine is very effective in relieving this pain. The usual dose is 200 mg three times daily but it can be doubled or even trebled. It is usually continued for a few weeks after the symptoms are relieved. In cases resistant to carbamazepine relief may be obtained by injection of the ganglion with phenol or by section of the trigeminal root, but this is rarely needed. Anaesthesia dolorosa is a rare sequel. These procedures are effective despite the fact that the primary pathological disturbance is located in the brain stem. The surgical measures do leave the patient with sensory loss over the face.

Facial Palsy and Deafness. Facial palsy, when isolated is likely to be regarded as a Bell's palsy, an error that may be reinforced when it clears in the course of a few weeks, which is the usual outcome. Often, there is sensory loss over the face and other evidence of the disease. Deafness is commoner than is generally appreciated but seldom severe enough to limit conversation.

Facial myokymia is a continuous rhythmic contraction of muscles which usually appears early in the disease. It clears in a few weeks but may recur.

Speech Disturbance. Dysphasia is rare but dysarthria is common. The slurred speech may make it very difficult for the patient to be understood or converse over the telephone. In the early stages it fluctuates, and it is often worse when the patient is physically exhausted. There is no satisfactory method of relieving this symptom. Speech therapy is disappointing. The bulbar muscles are seldom severely affected in this disease and problems of swallowing and inhalation of fluids arise only rarely.

Limb Weakness. This is a common symptom. In the lower limb it is usually associated with partial or complete foot drop and weakness of hip flexion. If the weakness is sufficient to cause the foot to be scraped along the ground, a support is helpful. The type of plastic support worn inside the shoe is seldom satisfactory except in the mildest cases. A toe spring and calliper is required, and the modern version is light but strong. Appliances designed to support the hip or knee are unsatisfactory and better avoided. A simple walking stick or stiff umbrella gives effective support and may prevent falls, although the patient is often reluctant to accept it. A tripod support or bipod frame gives greater support. A wheelchair may allow the patient to move independently.

The use of posterior column stimulation with an implanted extradural electrode to relieve paraparesis is currently under trial.

Sensory Symptoms. Paraesthesiae and numbness of the limbs and trunk are common. The sensation may be provoked by flexion of the neck when there is active disease of the cervical cord. No specific treatment is available but small doses of chlorpromazine may help and carbamazepine is sometimes advised but of doubtful value.

Ataxia. Cerebellar ataxia is particularly distressing and may make it difficult for the patient to walk at a stage when there is little other disability. A rubber tip on a walking stick is often helpful. This symptom is difficult to relieve and often persists. There is sensory ataxia when the posterior columns are involved in disease and this may remit. Truncal ataxia is sometimes prominent, particularly in an acute exacerbation of the disease.

In patients with severe intention tremor stereotaxic surgery has sometimes been advised. Our own limited experience of this technique has not been favourable.

Impotence. Impotence is a troublesome and often persistent symptom that may arise at an early stage in the disease. Sometimes it improves spontaneously but often it does not. Mechanical devices may help. In women there may be loss of vaginal sensation and loss of orgasm.

Spasticity. Increased resistance to passive movement is common in the limbs and trunk. Some patients who are very spastic have relatively good preservation of power. The severity of the spasticity varies in the early stages. It is aggravated by exposure to cold, distension of the bladder, and infection.

Such patients often develop *spasms* of the flexor, extensor, or adductor muscles. These may be provoked by movement or contact but also develop spontaneously. The spasms may be painful and are particularly troublesome in bed. Relief of the spasms can often be obtained from drugs, the most useful of which are diazepam, and baclophen. The dosage of some of these drugs is limited by associated sedative and hypnotic effects but this factor is less important at night (Table 11.2).

Table 11.2 Drugs used to Relieve Spasticity

Drug	*Initial dose daily*	*Effective dose range; daily*	*Other effects*
diazepam Valium	6 mg	6 to 100 mg	Somnolence is the limiting factor
baclophen Lioresal	30 mg	30 to 120 mg	Nausea, sedation, vertigo or flaccidity of limbs
mephanesin Myanesin	3 g	3 to 15 g	Nausea, confusion, ataxia, and diplopia
chlorpromazine Largactil	75 mg	75 to 200 mg	Sedation
dantrolene Dantrium	25 mg	200 to 800 mg gradual increase	Toxic hepatitis flaccidity

Spasticity is much more difficult to control than spasms. Assessment is also difficult because there is no satisfactory method of measuring spasticity. Some relief may be obtained with the drugs already mentioned with the dose increased gradually to the limit of tolerance. Baclophen, diazepam, and mephanesin are effective roughly in that order and should be used singly or in combination with chlorpromazine.

Severe spasticity can usually be relieved by injection of phenol intrathecally around the nerve root, or into the peripheral nerve. An alternative method is injection of alcohol at the motor point of the muscle. The intrathecal method is usually reserved for the patient with severe spasticity who is unable to walk. Occasionally, in selected cases, it may be used in those with severe spasticity who are mobile. It must be borne in mind that relief of spasticity may convert a stiff limb that functions as a prop into a flaccid one that will not support the patient. Bladder function is also an important consideration. When there is incontinence little effect is caused, but when the bladder is under voluntary control intrathecal phenol is better avoided. When these considerations are satisfied the use of intrathecal phenol may contribute substantially to the comfort of the patient by relieving spasm and allowing him to sit comfortably in a chair.

Intrathecal Phenol Injection. The technique recommended is that described by Liversedge and Maher (1960). It is important to explain to the patient what is proposed, making it clear that power in the limb will not be improved, and to allow time for full discussion before it is applied. The phenol solution is a 5 per cent concentration in glycerol and of higher specific gravity than spinal fluid. The dose is 1·0 to 2·0 ml. It is vitally important that it is not contaminated with water, otherwise the aqueous phenol may diffuse through the spinal canal.

The patient lies in the (left) lateral position and is prepared for lumbar puncture through the L2/3 space. The skin is anaesthetised. The patient is supported on pillows under the hip and shoulder and the trunk allowed to sag so that the point of injection is the lowest part of the spinal canal. The spinal needle is inserted and about 5 ml of fluid removed. A tuberculin syringe containing the phenol is attached (the viscosity of the solution is reduced if it is warmed slightly); 0·5 ml is injected and the patient is asked to report any sensation. Tingling in the thigh or around the (left) knee confirms that the level of injection is correct but this sensation may be absent. After a pause of a minute or two the injection is continued. At this stage there is often immediate relief of spasticity at the hip and knee. A decision is then made whether to withdraw the needle or to inject a further amount. The immediate relief is often greater than the final result. The knee-jerk is usually abolished and there may be sensory loss over the limb, but this often clears. The effect may be permanent, but if it is not the treatment can be repeated. The patient should remain in the lateral position for ten minutes after the injection. Afterwards the bladder function should be observed for a few days so that any tendency to retention of urine can be relieved. The other limb may then be treated in the same way.

Perineural Phenol Injection. The injection of phenol into peripheral nerve has been described by Halpern and Meelhuysen (1966). It can be applied to the upper as well as the lower limbs and is without effect on bladder function. An aqueous solution of phenol 2 or 3 per cent is used. A d.c.

stimulator is needed, and a 3 in (7·5 cm) spinal needle which is insulated with Teflon except at the tip. The cathode of the stimulator is connected to the needle and the nerve is approached as in performing a nerve block. The position is found at which a minimum current stimulus causes contraction of the muscle that is spastic. An injection of 0·1 to 5·0 ml is then given; 2 ml is usually sufficient. Satisfactory relief of spasticity and clonus is usually achieved. Paraesthesiae may cause trouble in some patients but usually settle in a few weeks. Numbness also clears after a few days.

Oedema. Patients who are relatively immobile and remain in the sitting position for long periods of time commonly develop oedema of the feet and legs. This is mainly due to impairment of the venous pump. The oedema clears when the feet are elevated. The swelling is often tolerated if its nature is explained. Diuretic therapy is not very effective and there is the further difficulty that it may make management of the bladder even more troublesome.

Bladder Management (*see also* Chapter 4). Bladder complications have important effects on the life of the patient with MS, and renal failure is a major cause of death. Such effects are usual when paraparesis is present but sometimes they become a dominant feature if the sacral part of the spinal cord is the site of disease.

Early symptoms include precipitancy of micturition and frequency. If infection is present there may be burning pain as well. Mild symptoms may be relieved by using atropine (0·6 mg) or probanthine (15 mg) several times during the day.

The urine should be examined microscopically and cultured: bacterial infection can then be treated with the appropriate antibiotic. In the early stages, catheterisation is probably better avoided since it almost always leads to infection. It may be needed if there is retention of urine or if a large residual volume is suspected.

Acute retention of urine may occur in an exacerbation of the disease. Catheterisation, and treatment of any infection will be needed. The situation often improves in the course of two or three weeks so that the patient is subsequently able to manage without a catheter. Injections of carbachol 0·5 mg subcutaneously may give relief. If retention persists transurethral bladder neck resection is sometimes performed. However, this is rarely required and such cases will need study by cystometrogram, micturating cystogram, and other urological methods.

Urinary incontinence in the male may be managed with a urinal drainage device or Paul's tubing if the patient is immobilised. In severe cases an indwelling catheter may be preferable. It should be changed every month and any infection treated.

In the female the management of incontinence is more difficult and no satisfactory drainage apparatus is available. In mild cases a pad may be sufficient, but in the more severe an indwelling catheter is usually needed. This may be of the Foley type and held in position by an inflated bulb. Leakage around the catheter may be troublesome.

The distress caused by incontinence or a catheter may lead to more radical treatments. Transplantation of the ureters into an ileal loop bladder presents special problems in these patients. Chronic infection is often present. If the surgical procedure is successful, spasm of the abdominal wall muscles may make it impossible to retain a plastic bag in position, and sometimes the final state may be worse than the situation it was designed to relieve. This procedure is contra-indicated in the presence of severe spasticity or muscle spasms, and there is the further difficulty that these features may become prominent at a later stage in the course of the disease.

Bowel Symptoms. Although disturbance of bowel motility and sphincter control are probably as common as bladder problems (and often co-exist) they generally cause less trouble to the patient. Chronic constipation and impaction of faeces must be avoided, liquid paraffin being valuable in prophylaxis. When incontinence develops, the possibility of impacted faeces must always be excluded by digital examination of the rectum.

Paroxysmal Dysfunction. Transient disturbances lasting a few seconds or minutes occasionally occur. There may be double vision, dysarthria, difficulty in swallowing, cerebellar disorder, or other clinical manifestation. This is sometimes reported when the patient is fatigued, or exposed to heat, but also happens spontaneously. These paroxysms are sometimes relieved by carbamazepine given by mouth in a dosage of 600 to 1800 mg daily for several weeks. There may be remissions.

Tonic attacks are brief, painful, unilateral, episodes that affect the face or limb and last only a few seconds. The clinical attack resembles tetany. Its nature is uncertain but it is probably due to subcortical epileptic discharge. Such attacks may precipitate in bouts over a period of days or weeks. Relief may be obtained by giving carbamazepine or another anticonvulsant.

Epileptic attacks are uncommon in the course of MS. They may be the presenting feature, take place during the course, or arise in the terminal phase. The commonest is a major convulsion, but temporal lobe episodes, Jacksonian attacks, or epilepsy partialis continua may occur.

The attacks usually settle over the course of a few months and often respond to anticonvulsant drugs.

General Management. The importance of making the patient independent cannot be over-emphasised and is the aim of rehabilitation. At this stage the patient is likely to be dependent on others, which may lead to bitterness and frustration. A situation may develop in which the spouse or other relation is almost fully occupied in caring for the patient over a long period of time, relief being obtained only when the patient is admitted to hospital. There is certainly a need to provide more facilities for short periods of institutional treatment to relieve the domestic burden. It is difficult to arrange for such patients to be admitted to general hospitals over holiday periods (when nursing staff is particularly scarce) and small hospitals could be more suitable for this purpose. Units for the young chronically disabled patient are now being developed. Those living at home may be supported by an attendance allowance.

Care of Skin. In the severely disabled patient the management of the skin and bladder becomes paramount. Prolonged pressure on the skin must be relieved and the patient in bed turned every two hours. Change in position is the most important factor in preventing bedsores. This simple truth, which is easily overlooked, accounts for the enormous difference in incidence of bedsores in various hospitals.

Psychological Disorder. It is often said that the patient with multiple sclerosis is euphoric, and it is fortunate when this attitude prevails. The factors that contribute to it are various and may include a cheerful disposition, lack of insight, deterioration in mental functions, and a determination to make the best of things.

The situation is not always so favourable and some patients become depressed. In the early stages this is most likely to be a reactive depression and phases of melancholia are almost inevitable. Severe depression may require treatment with drugs and supervision by a psychiatrist. Patients with advanced disease often show impairment of memory and intellectual functions. In some, this amounts to dementia and, occasionally, the effects are gross.

Appliances. A number of useful gadgets are available. In the home, bars fitted along walls and staircase, and wall handles help to support the patient. Zip fasteners are simpler to use than buttons. Holding devices are available to aid eating and drinking. Book rests and devices to turn the pages of a book can be obtained. A simple hoist ('Monkey pole') may enable the patient to move out of bed, and mechanical hoists are also obtainable although sometimes difficult to use. Absorbent pads are useful and sheepskin is probably the best material to place under the patient in bed. An electrically controlled ripple mattress will relieve constant pressure on the skin.

The Possum apparatus (patient operated selector mechanism) is electronically controlled and suitable for those with total or almost total paralysis of limbs. It can control such electrical devices as call system, heat, light, radio, and television, telephone and intercommunication system. It is available under the National Health Service but the high cost limits its general use.

A Functional Home. For the less severely disabled some other points may be considered. The patient should live on one level and preferably have a view from the window. Steps should be eliminated. Widening of doors may ease manipulation of a wheelchair. Underfloor heating is an advantage. In the bathroom and toilet, wallbars and a Remploy chair-bath with a shower tray in which it stands below floor level may allow independence. The avoidance of a large fluid intake in the evening (after 6 pm) may prevent bladder problems during the night. The electric blanket is useful and the patient is often more comfortable in a double rather than a single bed.

Transport. The problem of transporting the patient to work may be the limiting factor in determining whether he can continue. The combined use of a folding chair and a motorised vehicle may succeed if the patient is able to transfer himself from one to the other. His ability to drive will depend mainly on visual function and the degree of control of the limbs. If control of the upper limbs is satisfactory a conversion of a car to hand controls may be made. A Mobility Allowance is payable under the National Health Service (*see* Appendix 2).

Employment. Whenever possible the patient is encouraged to continue with his regular job or in similar work. If the work is physically demanding or requires special skills or fine manipulation this may not be possible. Clearly, a great deal will depend on the attitude of the employer, the length of time that the patient has been in the job, and the patient's resources for adaptation. Other important factors are personality, intelligence, and support from the family. When these factors are favourable the amount that can be achieved in the face of severe disability is sometimes remarkable. At the other extreme, regular work is clearly impossible. In the borderline group there is a tendency for the patient to be referred from one rehabilitation group to another when it is already clear from an objective assessment that training for other employment will not be possible.

Even when the assessment is just it may be very difficult to convince the patient that it is fair. A trial or work under supervision over a short period may be the best way of demonstrating the true situation. If competitive employment is not possible he may succeed in sheltered work such as is provided by Remploy. The patient with intellectual skills may be able to continue with his work at home, helped perhaps by tape recorder and typewriter.

Post-vaccinial and post-infective encephalomyelitis are discussed in Chapter 19.

12

Cerebral Vascular Disease

Under this heading we are concerned mainly with the effects of atherosclerosis and hypertension, which often lead to disability and death. The emphasis in treatment has shifted towards prevention. Control of hypertension has reduced the incidence of cerebral haemorrhage. Recognition of the transient ischaemic attack as a harbinger of a major stroke has led to attempts to control the factors that influence these minor episodes. Subarachnoid haemorrhage is often due to aneurysm, and when it is there is a major risk of a further attack. It is this tendency to recur that has stimulated surgical treatment of an aneurysm.

Systemic diseases may involve cerebral blood vessels, and although uncommon, their recognition is important in relation to medical treatment.

Despite recent advances in our understanding of the mechanisms of stroke, there remains a large population of disabled people who require rehabilitation and long-term care.

CEREBRAL HAEMORRHAGE

Cerebral haemorrhage will first be considered under the headings of primary subarachnoid haemorrhage and intracerebral haemorrhage. Extradural and subdural haematoma are particularly associated with head injury.

Primary subarachnoid haemorrhage is most often due to an aneurysm. There may be associated intracerebral bleeding, and spasm of cerebral arteries may lead to infarction. In primary intracerebral haemorrhage there is a strong correlation with systemic hypertension and blood may leak into the ventricle or subarachnoid space.

Primary Subarachnoid Haemorrhage. This may occur at any age, but is most often in a young adult. It develops suddenly with severe occipital headache, and coma may supervene within a few minutes. Signs of meningeal irritation are found, and there may be neurological deficit. Transient hypertension is common. Occasionally, the fundus shows subhyaloid haemorrhage or papilloedema.

The diagnosis is confirmed by lumbar puncture, which shows uniformly bloodstained fluid under raised pressure with yellow supernatant in the early stages. After a few days the fluid is yellow and clears after about three weeks.

When the diagnosis is established possible causes are considered. A cranial bruit suggests arteriovenous malformation. Persistent hypertension may be due to renal disease, coarctation of the aorta, or endocrine disorder (phaeochromocytoma). Pituitary apoplexy may cause a similar picture; the sella is then likely to be enlarged when seen in a lateral radiograph. Other causes include anticoagulant therapy, blood disorder, and drug interaction such as tyramine (cheese) and a monoamine oxidase inhibitor.

If the patient remains conscious survival is likely. Coma leads to death in about 30 per cent of cases and while coma persists the outcome remains uncertain. There is a high recurrence rate when aneurysm is the cause.

Two considerations determine management; intensive care following the incident and search for a cause. If an aneurysm or arteriovenous malformation is found, surgical treatment to prevent recurrence must be considered. The risk is greatest during the second week after the initial haemorrhage. Since the management is primarily a neurosurgical matter, the surgeon should be consulted at an early stage.

Intensive care in the acute stage is that required for coma or, if the patient is conscious, relief of pain. The irritable patient may settle after lumbar puncture and sometimes it is helpful to repeat it. The treatment is supportive and conservative at first and any attempt at radical surgery in the first 48 hours carries a prohibitively high mortality. It has been claimed that the administration of ε-aminocaproic acid, which inhibits fibrinolysis, reduces the risk of further haemorrhage. The dose is 0·1 g/kg given five times daily by slow intravenous infusion or by mouth. The effect is enhanced where there is renal failure. Dizziness, nausea, and diarrhoea may be caused, hence the advantage of this therapy is doubtful. Deepening of the coma or the development of focal signs may raise the possibility of haematoma, but the same signs can be due to cerebral ischaemia. The echo-encephalogram is helpful and the computerised axial tomogram will demonstrate haematoma or infarct and help to distinguish between them. In most cases it is better to avoid surgical treatment of a haematoma, but an expanding mass may occasionally require drainage in the acute stage. Surgical results are poor when the patient is in coma or has a gross neurological deficit.

After a day or two if the irritability has passed and the clinical condition stabilised with evidence of recovery of consciousness, the pursuit of the cause can continue. If aneurysm or arteriovenous malformation is suspected *and the patient is considered potentially fit for operation* arteriography is done. If arteriography is attempted in the first few hours the result is likely to be a poor demonstration of the vessels due to spasm. Persistent spasm may lead to death. In the elderly and those unfit for radical treatment there is little point in proceeding to arteriography. Both carotid arteries and the vertebro-basilar circulation are investigated because there may be more than one aneurysm and the first to be identified may not be responsible for the haemorrhage.

When an aneurysm has been demonstrated, the best surgical treatment is by direct approach, usually with a clip on the neck of the aneurysm. If this is not possible, the alternative of ligation of a main feeding vessel such as the carotid artery needs consideration when the aneurysm arises from it or is close to it. Use of the operating microscope has improved technique, and this is particularly valuable when the aneurysm is on the anterior communicating artery. Much skill is required in surgical treatment, and the result in favourable cases can be most satisfactory.

Usually, the patient is kept at rest for two to three weeks, active movement of the limbs being important to prevent thrombosis. Severe headache in the acute stage may justify powerful analgesics such as diamorphine 5 to 10 mg subcutaneously, and this may need to be repeated. Later it can be replaced by pentazocine and simpler analgesics.

There may be residual neurological signs, and sometimes there is epilepsy. It is an indication for anticonvulsant therapy, phenytoin being suitable. Occasionally, after recovery from the acute illness or at a much later stage, the patient shows mental deterioration due to low-tension hydrocephalus. This may be relieved by a shunt. Arteriovenous malformations may be amenable to surgical treatment if they are small. The prognosis without surgical treatment is better than for aneurysm, and recurrent haemorrhage milder.

Spinal Subarachnoid Haemorrhage. A rare disorder associated with severe pain in the back. It is usually due to an arteriovenous malformation of the spinal cord. The abnormal circulation is independent of the blood supply to the cord. Diagnosis is by myelography which shows a 'corkscrew' appearance in place of the normal smooth outline of the cord. Spinal arteriography can be performed using a catheter in the aorta to fill the branches. Usually, one main vessel is shown arising in the lower thoracic region. Surgical excision of the malformation may be possible. Sometimes a bruit is heard over the spine.

Intracerebral Haemorrhage. The differentiation of arterial occlusion from haemorrhage may be impossible from a clinical assessment. The onset of haemorrhage is abrupt and headache is common. Neurological deficit may evolve rapidly and hemiplegia is common. Systemic hypertension and left ventricular hypertrophy are often associated. In a doubtful case arteriography will confirm that the main arteries are patent, or demonstrate an expanding lesion. The computerised axial tomogram is helpful in differentiating haemorrhage and infarction. Haemorrhage is less permeable to X-ray.

The management is conservative with rest initially and control of hypertension. Surgical aspiration is rarely successful but aspiration of haematoma is sometimes performed when the patient is deteriorating and a large expanding mass has been shown by computerised axial tomogram or arteriography. Cerebellar haemorrhage is reported to respond well to this treatment but is uncommon. Such a patient is likely to present with unilateral cerebellar signs, headache, vertigo, severe vomiting, and raised intracranial pressure of rapid onset.

Extradural Haemorrhage (*see* Chapter 13). This haemorrhage is a complication of head injury, with rupture of the middle meningeal artery. It is likely to present within 48 hours of the injury. Impairment of consciousness is associated with dilatation of the pupil on the same side. The treatment is urgent surgical evacuation of the clot with occlusion of the artery.

Subdural Haematoma (*see* Chapter 13). This may develop as an acute haematoma following head injury or, more gradually, with fluctuating signs and headache evolving over a period of weeks. It is quite often bilateral. Treatment is surgical evacuation of the clot. When the haematoma has been present for several weeks a membrane may form around it.

Hypertensive Encephalopathy. The condition is most likely to arise in a patient with severe hypertension and renal disease or toxaemia of pregnancy. It presents with headache, convulsions, coma, cortical blindness and, sometimes, other neurological deficits. The distinction from cerebral haemorrhage may be difficult.

Emergency treatment is directed to the reduction of blood pressure, control of cerebral oedema, and anticonvulsant therapy. Diazoxide 300 mg i.v. given slowly will reduce blood pressure and can be repeated, or pentolinium 2 mg s.c. This is followed by an oral hypotensive regime. Intravenous diazepam may be useful to control convulsions, and dexamethasone 4 to 20 mg daily will control cerebral oedema.

Management of Hypertension. There is general agreement that hypertension is a factor in cerebrovascular disease and it is rational to control it when the diastolic pressure exceeds 100 mm. The risks of reducing the blood pressure have been exaggerated in the past. The possibility of a treatable cause will lead to consideration of renal disease, endocrine disease, or coarctation of the aorta. The importance of continued control of blood pressure must be stressed.

When no treatable cause is found the therapy will depend on the severity. In mild cases, a thiazide diuretic such as bendrofluazide 10 mg daily may be sufficient or combined with propranolol starting with 40 mg daily and increasing gradually to about 500 mg daily if tolerated. Methyldopa 250 mg three times daily can be combined with a diuretic and the dose may be increased to 2 g daily. If these fail, bethanidine 5 mg twice daily increased gradually to between 30 and 100 mg daily, or guanethidene 10 mg daily (single dose) increased every five days by 10 mg to between 30 and 100 mg daily, or debrisoquine 10 mg twice daily increased to 150 mg daily divided into three doses. Any of these may be combined with a diuretic, and potassium supplements will then be needed.

Postural hypotension is a troublesome feature and whenever possible the treatment should be instituted with the patient ambulant. Reduction in weight is advisable for the obese.

OCCLUSIVE VASCULAR DISEASE

Cerebral infarction may be associated with thrombosis or embolism and when an intracranial artery is occluded it is not possible to restore the arterial flow by surgical or medical treatment. Two factors have changed the management of occlusive vascular disease in recent years. The appreciation that occlusion or stenosis of the extracranial vessels (carotid and vertebral) are commonly present and the recognition of the transient ischaemic attack.

Transient Ischaemic Attack. This term implies a clinical episode in which neurological deficit develops and is sometimes severe but clears completely. The definition of the duration of the attack is somewhat arbitrary but one hour is often taken as the maximum. It may be much shorter and last only a few seconds. Transient ischaemic episodes are related particularly to occlusive disease but it is, of course, possible that a small haemorrhage might also cause brief and reversible effects. Haemodynamic crisis due to fall in local cerebral blood flow may be the cause in some cases. The most clearly demonstrated example of embolism arises in a patient with monocular visual loss in whom occlusion of retinal vessels can be seen to occur and later to clear, and a carotid bruit in the neck leads to the recognition of carotid stenosis on that side. It is then likely that platelet aggregates are detached from the stenosed area and pass to the eye and brain. It is certain that this process is much commoner than is generally recognised and only the more severe episodes cause clinical symptoms. Emboli may also arise in the heart in association with valvular disease, myxoma of the atrium, arrhythmia, or after cardiac infarction. The crucial question determining treatment and prognosis is whether the transient ischaemic attack is the prelude to more permanent effects. It has been shown that when transient ischaemic attacks develop in the territory of the carotid artery and its branches there is a serious risk of a major stroke within five years. In the vertebrobasilar territory the prognosis is less serious, and recovery from brainstem episodes may be substantial although cortical blindness or hemianopia usually persist.

Management. A full clinical appraisal of the patient, and particularly the cardiovascular system and peripheral circulation is the first step. If hypertension is present, its treatment becomes the dominant factor, and arteriography is not indicated unless there are signs of carotid stenosis. A localised bruit over the carotid artery may indicate stenosis but clears if occlusion supervenes. Before proceeding with arteriography (which remains the only reliable means of demonstrating stenosis) simpler screening tests should be carried out. The blood count may show anaemia or polycythaemia. A high sedimentation rate will raise the possibility of collagen disease. The chest radiograph and cardiograph are useful. The serological tests for syphilis are worth doing. The serum lipids and cholesterol and blood glucose may reveal predisposing factors.

Direct puncture for arteriography of the carotid artery carries some risk and aortography with catheterisation of the main vessels is safer. There is no purpose in detailed arteriography in the elderly and disabled or those shown clinically to have diffuse arterial disease or heart failure.

When systemic disease is found the treatment is directed towards it. If carotid occlusion is demonstrated, surgery is not usually feasible. If carotid stenosis is shown, what should be done, and the measures available have to be considered even before arteriography is done. The possible measures are surgical treatment of the stenosis or medical treatment with anticoagulant and antiplatelet regimes. It has to be admitted that the results are disappointing in general and sometimes little better than a supportive regime.

Surgical Treatment of Carotid Stenosis. Before this is attempted the surgeon will want to know the state of the other main vessels as revealed on aortography. The stenosed area may be cleared by endarterectomy, taking care to avoid allowing material to pass up the carotid artery; this has the disadvantage that it is likely to be followed by further deposition on the raw area. A by-pass procedure may be adopted and this requires clamping of the carotid artery while it is done.

Medical Management. Anticoagulant therapy has been widely used. We have been impressed in some cases when the use of anticoagulant has been associated with the cessation of a series of episodes, but the long-term effects are less satisfactory. There is some evidence that the disease has phases of activity, and clearly it would be appropriate to give treatment at that time, but there is no simple method of recognising activity except when clinical events are taking place. Platelet regimes are currently under trial. Aspirin may be used in a dose of 300 to 600 mg daily. Alternatives are sulphinpyrazole 400 to 800 mg daily and dipyridamole 400 mg/day. Intravenous rheomacrodex (Dextran 40) 200 ml/day is worth using after an acute episode if there is progression.

The duration of this therapy is difficult to determine and it is often hard to justify stopping the therapy. If the concept of phases of activity is accepted then treatment for a period of months may be rational.

While a full evaluation is awaited there is a tendency to use these regimes as the only positive line of treatment. The alternative, to await events, may well be disastrous but further episodes do happen despite careful therapy.

Anticoagulant Therapy. Heparin is the best anticoagulant but it must be given intravenously. A dose of 100 mg (10 000 units) every four to six hours is usually adequate to increase the clotting time to about 15 minutes. It can be neutralised with protamine.

Warfarin is the oral drug of choice and is readily absorbed. The initial dose is 40 mg. After 48 hours the prothrombin time is checked and a daily dose of 3 to 10 mg is usually required. It is more rapidly metabolised in the liver in patients on phenytoin.

Phenindione is an alternative but is not regularly absorbed and more likely to cause a hypersensitivity reaction. The usual dose is 200 mg initially, 100 mg on the second day, and an average of 100 mg daily, depending on the prothrombin time.

Subclavian Steal Syndrome. In this uncommon situation stenosis of the subclavian artery has the effect of causing reversal of blood flow in a vertebral artery so that the brain is actively deprived of blood. Studies of the natural history of this disorder are incomplete and sometimes the effect is temporary. In the usual type the pulse in the left arm is reduced and there is a bruit over the subclavian artery. Use of the left arm may cause pain or weakness or the patient may develop dizziness or other features associated with brain-stem ischaemia. Direct surgery to correct the arterial anomaly carries significant risk but the results of by-pass graft are encouraging.

Serum Cholesterol and Lipids in Relation to Treatment. In the uncommon condition of familial hypercholesterolaemia the use of drugs such as clofibrate by mouth in a dose of 1·5 to 2·0 g daily will lower the blood level and improve the prognosis.

A similar effect in lowering both blood cholesterol and triglyceride can also be seen in patients with vascular disease. However important these substances may be in pathogenesis, there is no definite evidence that the use of drugs of this type improves the outlook in cardiac or cerebral vascular disease. Clofibrate potentiates the action of anticoagulant drugs. It should be avoided in those with liver or kidney disease and during pregnancy.

The use of diets on the same basis is of unproved value although it would be generally agreed that reduction in weight is desirable for the obese.

Conclusions. The subject remains controversial and there is no clear evidence of the value of medical or surgical treatment. Enthusiasm for surgical treatment has not led to general acceptance of its advantages. We advise surgical treatment for isolated carotid stenosis when the patient is in good clinical condition. When transient ischaemic episodes recur we use an antiplatelet or anticoagulant regime, while awaiting the results of drug trials that are in progress. Antiplatelet regimes are unlikely to affect cholesterol emboli.

MANAGEMENT OF THE PROGRESSIVE STROKE

In most instances, occlusive vascular disease is manifest either as transient ischaemic episodes or a definitive stroke which does not progress, but occasionally the clinical state evolves over a period of days in a slow progression. The management is unsatisfactory and no firm advice can be given. Anticoagulant therapy is usually rejected for two reasons; if haemorrhage is a possible cause it is harmful, and if an infarct has developed there is a serious risk of haemorrhage into it. Arteriography is also risky when active disease is present. Rheomacrodex is worth considering. Corticosteroid therapy with dexamethasone 16 mg daily or glycerol 50 g in 500 ml of 5 per cent glucose daily for a week by intravenous infusion may be useful in the control of cerebral oedema in the acute stroke.

MANAGEMENT OF THE ESTABLISHED STROKE

So far the emphasis has been placed on warning signals that may be recognised as a prelude to a major stroke. It may be due to haemorrhage or infarction and is a common cause of both death and morbidity. In this section the less specific measures in management of the acute stroke and rehabilitation will be considered.

In the acute stage intensive care is needed. The airway must be cleared and maintained but assisted respiration is seldom justified. Feeding by nasogastric tube may be needed. The patient in coma will require the full routine of general care, frequent turning, catheterisation, and other supportive measures. Hypertension should be controlled, but it is better to avoid sudden falls in blood pressure. Recent cardiac infarction is sometimes the precipitating cause of a stroke, and arrhythmia or cardiac failure need treatment.

Passive movement of limbs is important in the early stages, but active movements are encouraged as soon as possible. After a few days an attempt at mobilisation can be made in the milder cases and even the more severely disabled. Exercises can then be directed towards the affected part. In the past much more attention has been given to motor deficits, but problems of speech, spatial orientation, and apraxia present an even greater challenge. The main value of intensive therapy is undoubtedly due to the cheerful and optimistic atmosphere created and the encouragement the patient receives. It is often difficult to evaluate the other aspects. Speech therapy, for example, may help but it is often felt that if the patient is capable of recovery of speech this will come naturally, and intensive therapy is not really needed.

The prognosis for recovery is good if there is improvement during the first few days or weeks. If no recovery has taken place after a month, there may still be improvement, but it is likely to be slow.

Rehabilitation after a stroke is designed to make the patient as independent as possible. A toe-spring caliper will control foot drop. A tripod, bipod frame, wheelchair, or motorised chair may help. Supporting bars in the bathroom and a 'monkey pole' over the bed are useful. An occupational therapist may visit the home and give advice.

Vascular Disease in Pregnancy, and the Contraceptive Pill. The occurrence of hemiplegia and other neurological deficit has long been known as an occasional event in the later stages of pregnancy. In some cases this is due to venous sinus thrombosis, and others are caused by arterial occlusion. The same may happen to women taking the contraceptive pill, and it is aggravated by a high oestrogen content. Arterial occlusion may be due to embolism. Migraine may be made worse by the contraceptive pill, but this does not always happen. Other predisposing factors such as hypertension, collagen disease (SLE) increase the risk and the contraceptive pill is better avoided in these patients. The occurrence of a mild stroke, focal features associated with migraine, or retinal vascular disorders are indications to stop the contraceptive pill.

Cortical Venous Thrombosis. Cortical thrombophlebitis has been mentioned in relation to intracranial infection. Thrombosis of venous sinuses may also occur after head injury and in systemic diseases. Epilepsy is an indication for anticonvulsant therapy. The value of anticoagulant therapy is not clear and it has little place in the presence of infection.

Cerebral Blood Flow and Drugs. Alteration in cerebral blood flow can be demonstrated in patients with cerebral artery occlusion or arteriosclerosis. Drug therapy can be shown to modify this, but the dynamic state is complicated and cerebral autoregulation is an important consideration. The inhalation of 5 per cent carbon dioxide has been advised in the past as a vasodilator after a stroke. This is now regarded as potentially harmful as it may actually divert blood from the ischaemic area to other parts of the brain. The same problem arises with vasodilator drugs such as papaverine and tolazoline.

Other drugs have been reported to improve cerebral metabolism in a geriatric population, but the advantages are marginal. Recent work on cerebral blood flow has contributed to our understanding of the mechanism of stroke, but has not yet helped in routine management.

13

Head Injuries

In an increasingly industrialised and urbanised environment the number of hospital admissions for head injury is rising. The criteria for admission of minor head injuries may vary from district to district, but a history of unconsciousness, vomiting after head injury, and any degree of mental confusion are reasons for admission. As there are multiple injuries in approximately 50 per cent of casualties with head injuries, other factors may govern the admission. The small number of specialised Head Injury Units means that many patients are admitted to general wards in a district hospital. Road accidents are the commonest cause, and in industrialised areas injuries at work are the second major factor. The improvement in survival due to advances in nursing care and improved management of early complications has left a residue of brain-damaged patients requiring long-term care.

EARLY ASSESSMENT

Initial contact with a patient with head injury may be at the work site, the roadside, or in a casualty department. The head injury itself may be minor, with no loss of consciousness, vomiting or amnesia. Attention is then directed to any associated injuries. If the patient is conscious on arrival in casualty, it may be possible to obtain an account of the accident, but in many instances this is impossible. It is important to know whether consciousness was lost immediately or whether there was deterioration in level of consciousness following a lucid interval. The patient's general condition must be assessed. Shock due to blood loss must be corrected as soon as possible. This is usually due to an associated injury.

When it has been decided that the major problem is a head injury a basic neurological assessment must be made. The level of consciousness is determined. Coma is a state in which there is no conscious mental response to the external or internal environment. There is no response to pinprick. Semicoma indicates a condition of unconsciousness but with response to painful stimuli, including facial movements. Confusion indicates clouding of consciousness of varying severity. In the mildest form there is confusion, but conversation can take place. In severe confusion the patient will respond only to occasional simple commands. Changes in the level of consciousness must be carefully recorded. The pulse may be feeble and rapid due to shock or terminal head injury. If there is cerebral compresson it may slow. A rise in blood pressure may indicate cerebral compression or anoxia. The respiratory pattern may be rapid and deep in brain stem damage or respiratory patterns may develop such as Cheyne-Stokes respiration. The pupils may be normal, small or dilated. Unilateral dilation of the pupil may indicate tentorial herniation or direct trauma to the oculomotor nerve.

Inspection of the skull and scalp is important. An extensive scalp wound may indicate a compound penetrating injury. Bleeding from the ears or nose may be associated with middle or anterior fossa fractures.

One of the most important factors in early survival from a severe head injury is the maintenance of a proper airway. Mechanical difficulty in breathing may be the result of chest injuries, and injuries to the face, jaws, and tongue may be involved. If it is impossible to maintain satisfactory respiration with an airway, endotracheal intubation is required. This is acceptable for a period of several days but beyond this stage a tracheostomy is necessary. This has an advantage in reducing the dead space and making suction easier.

EARLY MANAGEMENT AND THE MANAGEMENT OF THE UNCONSCIOUS PATIENT

Early observation of head injuries should begin when the patient is first seen. Regular observations of the pulse, pupil size and response, and respiratory pattern should be made, usually at fifteen minute intervals until the clinical state is stable. Changes in these signs are of importance as they may indicate cerebral compression. Headache may persist for some time and, provided there are no other problems, need not require prolonged bedrest.

The nursing of an unconscious patient requires turning at two-hourly intervals. This is best recorded on a turn chart which is initialled by the nurses involved at the appropriate time. Failure to turn will result in pressure sores.

Patients who are irritable and restless while recovering consciousness may prove difficult to nurse. On the whole, sedation should be avoided but the use of a phenothiazine such as chlorpromazine in 50 mg doses may help. These patients are not easily confined to bed by using cot sides and in many instances they may be nursed on a mattress on the floor. Cot sides with a net over the top are another alternative.

Nutrition and the maintenance of a reasonable fluid intake must be continued. In an unconscious patient, a nasogastric tube is used and hourly fluids given, together with a liquid diet. The urinary output must be measured. If the patient is unconscious, incontinence will be a problem. In the female this requires catheterisation; in the male an appropriately placed urinal or a piece of tubing attached to the penis and connected to an appropriate receptacle may suffice. An accurate fluid balance chart must be maintained and the patient's blood urea and electrolytes monitored. The development of diabetes insipidus can then be diagnosed.

Surgical Procedures. During the early stage, obvious surgical procedures may be necessary. Scalp wounds should be sutured in an operating theatre when the presence of a penetrating brain wound has been excluded. This possibility is the main reason against suturing scalp wounds in an unconscious patient in the casualty department.

If a depressed fracture of the skull is present it must be decided whether to elevate it or not. One of the main reasons for doing so is the high incidence of epilepsy following depressed skull fractures. This is much greater when the dura has been breached. In this instance loose spicules of bone penetrating the brain should be removed and the fracture elevated.

Severe Brain Damage. The patient who is deeply unconscious from the time of the accident frequently has irreversible brain stem damage. The term concussion has been applied to patients who lose consciousness briefly and appear confused or amnesic but fully recover. This represents the mild end of a spectrum which extends to widespread neuronal dysfunction in the brain stem with resultant brain stem failure.

Decerebrate posturing frequently occurs in the context of severe brain injury. This may be accompanied by attacks of shivering and hyperpyrexia. In decerebrate postures the arms may be flexed, adducted and internally rotated, being extended at the elbow and flexed at the wrist and fingers. The legs are extended and the feet plantar flexed. Sometimes the arms are adducted and flexed across the body. These postures may be symmetrical or unilateral or asymmetrical. They may be episodic and associated with sweating and deepening respiration. The use of a cocktail containing 50 mg of pethidine, 50 mg of chlorpromazine and 25 mg of promethazine intramuscularly helps to reduce the shivering, posturing, and hyperpyrexia. Although these signs indicate severe neuronal dysfunction, there may be remarkable degrees of recovery in long-term survivors.

SPECIFIC EARLY COMPLICATIONS

The number of sophisticated investigations carried out on brain-damaged patients varies from centre to centre. It is normally possible to recognise deterioration due to cerebral compression, and then burr holes are the quickest way of exploring the problem. An echo-encephalogram may show a central shift. Angiography is sometimes utilised but the degree of usage varies. It has probably been over-used in patients who remain deeply unconscious from the time of the head injury. Computerised transverse axial tomography of the brain is a major advancement in the assessment of head injuries. One limiting factor is the restlessness of the patient. This investigation will reveal collections of blood and their site and demonstrate oedema. Air not seen on plain X-rays may be demonstrated. The real problem with this major diagnostic advance is how to utilise the information it provides. The presence of a small intracerebral haematoma or subdural haematoma does not necessarily mean operative treatment is required. The relevance of these findings to the patient's clinical status must be assessed. The other problem is the limited availability of the technique.

Seizures. Early seizures can be defined as taking place in the first week after head injury. Such attacks predispose the patient to the development of late post-traumatic epilepsy. The majority of early fits appear in the first 24 hours and are generalised or focal motor attacks. Temporal lobe attacks are seldom seen in the first week. Early epileptic fits should be treated with anticonvulsants, and phenytoin is suitable. Status epilepticus is best treated with intravenous diazepam or clonazepam.

Extradural Haematoma. The diagnosis of this is an urgent matter. A skull fracture in the region of the middle meningeal artery may act as a pointer. It should be suspected in any patient with a deteriorating level of consciousness and a unilateral dilated pupil following head injury. The clinical picture may evolve over minutes. In the case of a venous extradural haematoma the presentation is delayed several days. A lucid interval may have intervened. The treatment is surgical evacuation and control of the bleeding point. The prognosis is good if diagnosed early. Late diagnosis may be associated with irreversible brain damage, particularly in the elderly.

Subdural Haematoma. In acute subdural haematoma the patient will present with clinical features of cerebral compression if the haematoma is significant. The best way of distinguishing subdural, extradural, and intracranial haematomas is by computerised tomography. The existence of a small subdural haematoma does not necessarily constitute a reason for surgery. The important clinical problem may be widespread neuronal damage or cerebral oedema. Acute subdural haematoma carries a poor prognosis despite surgical intervention.

Chronic subdural haematoma presents as a fluctuating confusional state with or without papilloedema, sometimes with a history of a trivial head injury. Such patients are investigated as if a space-occupying lesion of unknown cause was present. The results of surgical evacuation are good unless the diagnosis is delayed and a chronic adherent membrane has formed.

Intracerebral Haematoma. Cerebral compression due to an intracerebral haematoma presents with a deteriorating level of consciousness and altering focal neurological signs. The mere presence of an intracerebral haematoma does not necessarily indicate it is the cause of clinical deterioration. A diagnosis may be made by angiography or computerised axial tomography.

Traumatic Subarachnoid Haemorrhage. Microscopic blood may be present in the CSF even if the injury is not severe. More marked haemorrhage will cause meningeal irritation and a lumbar puncture should be performed to exclude meningitis.

Cerebral Oedema. The patient whose conscious level is deteriorating and who is comatose should receive dexamethasone 4 mg 6-hourly but the possibility of a haematoma must be kept in mind. Monitoring the intraventricular pressure may be helpful. Computerised tomography of the brain will distinguish between haematoma and oedema.

Fat Embolism. This usually occurs within the first seventy-two hours following an injury. There is a fracture of a large bone such as the femur. The embolism causes multiple signs and symptoms. Fat may appear in the urine. Permanent damage may result, although in many instances there is a good recovery. There is no specific treatment. Dexamethasone may be used for accompanying cerebral oedema.

Brain Stem Failure. This is a grave complication. Spontaneous respiration ceases or becomes irregular and there is a drop in blood pressure. The only way to keep such patients alive is with assisted respiration. Prolonged respiratory management is not justified. It is necessary to explain to the relatives that there is no hope of recovery and that life is being maintained by artificial means. Provided adequate explanation is given, there is usually no difficulty in convincing the relatives that the respirator should be switched off. Patients dying in this way may have suitable kidneys for transplantation.

LATE SEQUELAE

The presence of long-term complications is assessed after the acute period is over. This can be regarded as the end of post-traumatic amnesia or when there is no reasonable prospect of recovery of normal consciousness. If this is over 24 hours the patient has had a severe head injury. The post-traumatic amnesia may last for months after severe injuries.

Persistent Vegetative State. This term was proposed by Jennett and Plum. It refers to patients who survive a severe brain injury for months or years with no evidence of recovery of higher cerebral function. Those in coma tend to improve after a few weeks but never develop any purposeful activity. Some have akinetic mutism and lie immobile but apparently alert. The term coma vigile refers to a similar condition. These patients require tube feeding, catheterisation, and constant nursing care. Early measures adopted to preserve life has produced a group of helpless patients who have no conscious existence. The persistent vegetative state may be caused by diffuse white matter damage as described by Strich.

The 'locked-in-syndrome' refers to a de-efferented state due to a lesion in the base of the pons sparing the tegmentum. The patient is tetraplegic and aphonic. He may be mistakenly regarded as having akinetic mutism. Communication can be carried out by blinking or vertical eye movements. The pathological basis is usually vascular or demyelinating.

Intellectual Deterioration. This is usual after severe head injuries. A previously intelligent individual may still be able to return to his former job but cerebral reserve is reduced and in a profession such as teaching the level of ability may be reduced. Psychometry provides a measurement of intellectual status. There is no specific treatment. Improvement may continue for up to two years following the injury.

Industrial rehabilitation may assist in training for a simpler job. Associated physical defects may affect the rehabilitation programme. A full assessment for independent daily living and job suitability should be carried out by an occupational therapist. Gross brain damage leaves the patient incapable of independent existence and continuous care is required. This is best managed at home. The only other facilities are in long-stay psychiatric wards, mental subnormality hospitals, and units for the young chronic disabled.

Personality Change. This is common after a severe head injury and usually associated with intellectual deterioration. Altered affect, emotional lability, uninhibited behaviour with sexual deviation, hyposexuality and aggressive outbursts occur. There is no specific treatment. In extreme cases behaviour may be unacceptable and require in-patient care. Phenothiazines may be helpful in controlling aggression and hyperactivity but, in general, the value of drugs is limited and environmental factors are more important.

Cranial Nerve Palsies. In the assessment of cranial nerve palsies it should be remembered that they have occurred in the acute stage and their assessment is left until later. They do not require specific treatment.

Anosmia due to olfactory nerve damage may recover over a few months but is often permanent. It destroys smell sensation and food appreciation. Gas appliances should be avoided. The enjoyment of previously pleasant olfactory experiences is lost. Anosmia may follow minor head injuries particularly to the occiput.

The optic nerve may be damaged by blows near the orbit. Visual failure and optic atrophy occur. This is permanent. Ocular nerve palsies may be due to fractures near the orbit or skull base. They may improve spontaneously. If diplopia persists for more than six months, ophthalmic surgery or the use of prisms may help.

Other cranial nerve disorders include the trigeminal, facial, auditory and vagus nerves, and no specific treatment is available apart from consideration of a cosmetic operation to improve facial appearances at a later stage.

Other Focal Neurological Defects. Higher function disorders such as dysphasia, dysarthria, spasticity or ataxia with or without weakness in one or more limbs may occur. Dysphasia should be treated by a speech therapist and slow and satisfactory recovery may come about over a period of years in severe cases.

Spasticity can sometimes be reduced by using dantrolene (page 120). The dose schedule is variable and several weeks may be required to stabilise the drug dosage. Baclofen may help. Diazepam is also used in some patients. Physiotherapy at an early stage reduces contractures but even with prolonged physiotherapy little improvement is seen in severe cases.

Ataxia is generally very disabling. Severe truncal or gait ataxia causes difficulty in sitting and the patient may be unable to walk unaided. In less severe degrees of gait ataxia, a rubber-tipped walking stick may help. Severe intention tremor involving one arm can only be overcome by learning to use the other arm.

Anticonvulsants after Head Injury. The overall incidence of epilepsy after head injury is about 5 per cent. Attacks during the first week (early epilepsy) are more liable in those with acute haematoma, in adults with prolonged post-traumatic amnesia, in children (and to a lesser degree adults) with depressed fracture, and in those with focal signs of brain damage. Early epilepsy predisposes to late epilepsy. The risk of late epilepsy developing becomes progressively less as the time interval from the injury increases and is significantly reduced after one year (Jennett).

The question arises, should anticonvulsant therapy be given as a routine to some or all head injuries, and for how long should it be continued? The value of such therapy is unproved, and controlled trials are awaited. Controversy centres around the problem of whether a solitary fit is harmful and may itself predispose to the development of an epileptic focus; if that is accepted as a serious risk, the case for routine administration of anticonvulsants is strengthened.

In favour of anticonvulsant therapy is the general belief that it will prevent the development of epilepsy; it is not a bar to driving in Britain. Against such therapy as a routine it will be noted that this would involve giving drugs to many patients who do not need them. It would be difficult to persuade some patients to continue with the therapy over a long period and irregular therapy is worse than none. It would probably modify the natural history and so make assessment of prognosis difficult or impossible.

In the absence of clear evidence, our own view is that the routine use of anticonvulsants is not justified. There is a case for regular therapy when a major predisposing factor is present, otherwise we would advise initiation of therapy after a definite fit. Once therapy has been started, we see little justification for stopping it in less than two years.

The Post-traumatic Syndrome (*see* Chapter 3). This consists of headache, dizziness and poor memory persisting for a considerable time after a head injury, which is frequently a minor one. There is some controversy with regard to the nature of this syndrome. One viewpoint is that the symptoms are the result of a compensation neurosis and only settle when compensation is provided. An important argument against this view is that similar symptoms occur in patients following minor head injuries where no compensation is involved.

It has been demonstrated that following a minor head injury, there may be vertigo which persists for as long as two years. In patients complaining of post-traumatic vertigo after minor head injuries, it is possible to induce positional nystagmus in some instances. Such patients may also complain of headache, although dizziness is the predominant symptom.

It has been pointed out that following minor injuries some people become depressed and anxious. Their symptoms are genuine and attributable to the accident and not the result of compensation neurosis. There is no doubt that this does happen, and treatment with diazepam or, if warranted, tricyclic antidepressants will alleviate the symptoms.

In conclusion, the post-traumatic syndrome has no single cause and each patient has to be evaluated individually. A high proportion of medico-legal cases in a series of patients studied tends to give rise to a false impression that all patients have a compensation neurosis. Although this applies in some instances it is by no means the only cause of the post-traumatic syndrome and organic or genuine psychiatric illness may be relevant.

ELECTRICAL INJURY TO THE BRAIN

This form of brain injury produces chromatolysis of ganglion cells and dilatation of the perivascular spaces. Petechial haemorrhages and disruption of large blood vessels occur. Fragmentation of peripheral nerve axons and burns on the skin may be present.

Damage may be due to the heat generated as in lightning or due to direct application of current to the skull. There is frequently loss of consciousness. Hallucinations and bizzarre sensory symptoms together with motor weakness may be present. The effects of electrocution are complex but artificial respiration and cardiac massage may be life saving. The use of dexamethasone is of value in reducing cerebral oedema.

14

Cerebral Tumours

The treatment of cerebral tumours is generally regarded as a surgical matter, and there can be few more satisfactory measures than the complete removal of a benign intracranial mass. Unfortunately, benign intracranial tumours are relatively uncommon and the surgical results in treatment of malignant and metastic tumour are poor. Recent advances in neuroradiology have increased the accuracy of diagnosis based on clinical findings and radiology. A biopsy is needed in the majority of cases. The best management of the individual patient must take account of the general health, life expectancy, and likely outcome of the proposed treatment in terms of the quality of life as well as the technical aspects of therapy.

Clinical Presentation. Tumours involving the cerebral hemispheres are likely to present with epilepsy, and progressive motor or sensory deficit on the opposite side. Frontal or temporal tumours may produce psychiatric symptoms and may reach a large size before they are recognised; epilepsy may lead to earlier diagnosis.

Progressive visual failure not attributable to glaucoma or other eye disease may be due to compression of the visual pathway by a meningioma, cranio-pharyngioma, or other tumour.

Posterior fossa tumours present with headache, papilloedema, and cerebellar signs.

Cerebral tumours must be distinguished from haematoma and abscess as well as occlusive vascular disease. Haematoma is likely to follow trauma but there may not be a history of injury. Cerebral infarction is usually abrupt in onset but can be confused with tumour, and both may show temporary clinical improvement.

Investigations. A search must be made for a primary tumour outside the nervous system and a chest radiograph is always needed. Plain radiographs of the skull, an EEG, echo-encephalogram and isotope brain scan are useful in preliminary assessment. The echo-encephalogram will demonstrate displacement of the midline.

The most useful investigation is the computerised axial tomogram. This is a non-invasive procedure which depends on alteration in tissue density and provides an anatomical section of the brain.

Alternative radiological methods include arteriography, and contrast studies using air or Myodil to demonstrate the ventricles. If the signs indicate a hemisphere lesion, a carotid arteriogram may be helpful and is safe even if the intracranial pressure is raised. The vessels may be displaced, and from this the location of a tumour mass and size of the lateral ventricle can be inferred.

Air encephalography should be avoided in patients with suspected intracranial hypertension or posterior fossa tumour. Air ventriculography requires a burr hole and the air is then injected into the ventricle. Myodil ventriculography is particularly valuable in showing lesions of the posterior fossa that may displace the aqueduct and fourth ventricle. Vertebral arteriography also has a place in the investigation of abnormalities of the posterior fossa.

Management of Cerebral Oedema and Intracranial Hypertension. Temporary relief can be obtained by intravenous infusion of mannitol 20 per cent using 200 to 500 ml over a period of twenty minutes. The osmotic diuresis which follows may lead to dehydration and electrolyte disturbance. Brain oedema can be controlled most effectively with corticosteroids. In urgent situations dexamethasone 8 mg may be injected intravenously. This may be followed by oral dexamethasone (4 to 16 mg daily) which leads to reduction of oedema and resolution of papilloedema. The duration of this effect is unpredictable, but it may last for several months if the drug is continued. Dexamethasone should be reserved for specific purposes. It should not be given before a policy of treatment has been decided or used to defer a surgical consultation. If surgical operation is planned it may be useful preoperatively, and is then continued afterwards. When removal of a tumour is impossible, dexamethasone may be a very useful symptomatic treatment, and allow the patient relief of headache. Caution is needed when there is infection, a history of peptic ulcer, or psychotic features which may be aggravated by corticosteroids.

Benign Intracranial Hypertension. A small proportion of the patients who present with raised intracranial pressure show no evidence of an intracranial mass or other cause. A few of them have endocrine disease or are related to reduction in dosage of corticosteroid therapy. Occasional cases are attributable to nalidixic acid, or tetracycline in infants. The remainder form a group that can only be identified after investigation. The key is usually the computerised axial tomogram or air ventriculogram which show normal or small ventricles in normal position. The condition is commonest in obese young women, but is also found in males and in older patients.

There is a danger of visual failure. Control of the intracranial pressure may be brought about by means of corticosteroid therapy (dexamethasone) or surgical (usually subtemporal) decompression. Repeated lumbar puncture is not recommended. Careful supervision is essential. The development of any focal neurological signs is a signal for further investigation. The condition may resolve over a period of a year or two but sometimes persists for longer. Withdrawal of dexamethasone must be gradual.

Metastatic Tumours. When there is a primary tumour in the lung, breast, or other tissue it is highly probable that an associated cerebral tumour is metastatic. This cannot always be assumed, and special care is needed if the primary mass has been removed several years previously and there is no other evidence of metastasis. When several discrete masses can be shown by isotope scan or other method, the diagnosis is much easier. It is doubtful whether surgical excision of metastases should be attempted, for results are poor. Excision is usually impracticable if there is more than one mass, or if a vital structure is involved. The question of excision of solitary masses is debatable and although a few reports of long survival are found in the literature, they are rare. The use of dexamethasone is recommended (page 147) and there may be rapid resolution of the physical signs. Radiotherapy is sometimes worthwhile, particularly if a tumour elsewhere has been shown to respond.

TUMOURS INVOLVING THE CEREBRAL HEMISPHERE

The main problem here is the differentiation of metastases from meningiomas and gliomas. Plain radiographs of the skull are abnormal in 50 per cent of meningiomas, and may show erosion, sclerosis, or altered vascular markings. The isotope scan may show multiple areas of uptake which favours metastases, and it is almost always positive in a meningioma. The location is significant because most meningiomas are over the convexity, parasagittal, or along the sphenoidal ridge. The computerised axial tomogram also may reveal multiple lesions, show the clear demarcation of a meningioma, and give a measure of radiological density. Carotid arteriography may show vessels passing to a meningioma from the external carotid system, a tumour blush, and displacement of intracranial vessels. With gliomas, an avascular area may be seen or a complex of new vessels. Biopsy will usually be needed to confirm the diagnosis and is best carried out at a craniotomy. Burr-hole biopsy may cause a sudden deterioration in the condition of the patient. Oedema is sometimes the reason for a meningioma being overlooked.

Meningiomas. These tumours are benign but may infiltrate the calvarium. The elective sites are shown in Table 14.1. They form about 15 per cent of all intracranial tumours.

Table 14.1. Elective Sites for Meningiomas

	%
Parasagittal and falx	30
Convexity	18
Sphenoidal ridge	18
Posterior fossa	10
Suprasellar	5
Olfactory groove and subfrontal	5
Subtemporal	5
Intraventricular	2
Other	7

A convexity meningioma tends to present with epilepsy, followed by raised intracranial pressure and then focal signs. The tumour can usually be removed, but may be vascular. Operative mortality is about 10 per cent.

A parasagittal meningioma often causes headache. Anteriorly placed tumours may lead to mental changes. Sometimes there is frontal incontinence. Epilepsy may be the presenting feature with focal attacks starting in the opposite foot. Foot drop and limb weakness may develop, and sensory loss. Posterior tumours produce homonymous hemianopia. Surgical removal of a parasagittal meningioma is difficult. Haemorrhage may cause death, and attachment to the sinus may make it impossible to remove the tumour completely. Operative mortality depends on the attitude of the surgeon towards attempting complete removal, and is about 25 per cent.

A sphenoidal ridge meningioma may present with visual failure, proptosis, or epilepsy (often of temporal lobe type). Plain radiographs often show erosion of bone. Surgical removal is difficult and operative mortality about 20 per cent.

If the meningioma is removed completely the outlook is good. Even when the tumour is not completely excised, growth may continue very slowly. There is recurrence sometimes. The value of radiotherapy is doubtful.

Gliomas. Gliomas are the commonest primary intracranial tumours and the range of malignancy is wide. Radical excision is probably impossible as there is no clear edge to the tumour which has usually infiltrated before diagnosis. The histological findings give some guide to prognosis. Multinucleate giant cell tumours (glioblastoma multiforme) are rapid-growing and not controlled by therapy so that the prognosis is poor. Astrocytomas show wide variation in malignancy and some tumours evolve slowly over many years. Excision is sometimes attempted if the mass is large and located in the non-dominant frontal or temporal lobe, which helps decompression. The oligodendroglioma is uncommon and may evolve slowly over many years.

Surgical treatment is of limited value and there is no effective therapy. Dexamethasone 4 to 20 mg daily will control the intracranial pressure for a limited period.

POSTERIOR FOSSA TUMOURS

A meningioma may arise in the posterior fossa and then usually presents with raised intracranial pressure. The acoustic neuroma is benign and amenable to surgery. Gliomas are relatively uncommon in the posterior fossa, the commonest primary tumour being the medulloblastoma in children.

Acoustic Neuroma. The early diagnosis of acoustic neuroma is difficult. This is partly because the early symptoms may be ignored by the patient, but tinnitus, deafness, and vertigo are common symptoms in other disorders of the auditory apparatus. Early diagnosis depends on awareness, expert assessment by an audiologist, special radiographs of the internal auditory meatus and Myodil meatography.

The definitive treatment is surgical. If the tumour is diagnosed when it is small, removal by a translabyrinthine approach (House) may be possible, and carries minimal risk. Much more frequently the diagnosis is reached late and this method is then impracticable. Excision of a large mass carries serious risks and complications. Death may result from infarction of the brain stem. Cerebellar or brain stem deficit may be made worse. Deafness and vestibular loss on the affected side are often present before operation, and persist afterwards. Usually there is a facial palsy as well.

A follow-up study of 130 patients seen three years after operation (Mackenzie 1965) showed that half had returned to full activity and pointed out that a lot depends on the courage and determination of the patient. Unilateral deafness causes difficulties in crowds or in traffic, and in localising sounds. Facial paralysis was a serious disability, particularly for women, and procedures such as facio-glossopharyngeal or facio-hypoglossal anastomosis can help. Facial numbness, clumsiness of the arm, and unsteadiness in walking were common problems. Vertigo, as opposed to unsteadiness, was rare.

Intracapsular removal carries a mortality of 10 to 20 per cent. Recurrent operations carry even greater risk, with a mortality approaching 50 per cent at five years. In the young patient, extracapsular (total) excision may be the treatment of choice, but in the elderly there are more complications. Sufficient has been said of the morbidity and mortality to show the excision of these benign tumours is often not straightforward. However, it does offer the best hope of arresting the progression of the condition. In those of advanced age it should, perhaps, be avoided. Partial excision is advised by some surgeons. The outlook after operation is much better when the tumour is small.

Glioma of the Brain Stem. This is uncommon and is most often found in children. It presents with multiple cranial nerve palsies. Biopsy is difficult and often better avoided. The diagnosis is then based on the clinical findings and Myodil ventriculography which shows displacement of the aqueduct. Radiotherapy is the treatment of choice and may arrest progress, but the effect is usually temporary.

Medulloblastoma of the Cerebellum. Medulloblastoma is found most often in children between 5 and 10 years old. It evolves as a midline mass arising from the vermis. In the adult it is more often seen in the cerebellar hemisphere. Surgical exploration is usually needed to confirm the nature of the tumour. Radiotherapy is the treatment of choice and must include the whole spinal canal so that seeding of the tumour through the spinal fluid is controlled. The five-year survival rate is about 30 per cent.

Cerebellar Astrocytoma in Children. This may be seen in the second decade of life and presents with ataxia and raised intracranial pressure. Surgical excision may be possible, and the results are often favourable.

The mass may be cystic.

In *ependymoma of the fourth ventricle* excision is often impossible but radiotherapy is worthwhile. There may be seeding of the tumour within the spinal canal.

Haemangioblastoma of the Cerebellum. Although one of the most rewarding tumours from the surgical point of view, early diagnosis may be difficult. The tumour consists of a small vascular mass with a cyst that may be filled with blood. It may present with ataxia and raised intracranial pressure, but in the early stages vertigo and vomiting may be prominent. Surgical excision is usually possible, and the long-term results are very favourable. Occasionally there is recurrence.

Vertebral arteriography may be helpful in diagnosis. Sometimes similar tumours are present in the retina, spinal canal, lung, liver, pancreas or other organs (Lindau's disease). Polycythaemia is found in a small proportion. Radiotherapy is useful if the tumour is large, vascular, and not amenable to surgery.

Chordoma. Tumour of the notochord may arise in childhood or later. It may be in the region of the brain stem, posterior fossa, or, most commonly, the sacrum. Surgical excision often presents considerable technical problems and the tumour is not sensitive to radiotherapy.

INTRAVENTRICULAR TUMOURS

Tumours within the ventricular system are relatively uncommon. A paraventricular glioma may invade the ventricles and a craniopharyngioma sometimes spreads to the anterior part of the third ventricle. Those that arise within the ventricles include glioma, meningioma, choroid plexus papilloma, epidermoid, and colloid cyst of the third ventricle.

Tumours in this situation may reach a large size before they cause symptoms. The usual presentation is raised intracranial pressure; other features are likely to be due to irritation of, or pressure upon, surrounding structures.

A choroid plexus papilloma is usually in the lateral ventricle, rarely malignant, and met with in children as well as adults. The tumour secretes cerebrospinal fluid. In the infant it may present as hydrocephalus—often in the second year of life—and sometimes accompanied by papilloedema.

Colloid cyst of the third ventricle is often located near to the foramen of Munro. It causes raised intracranial pressure and episodic weakness of the legs. The onset of symptoms may be abrupt and there may be dementia and features of hypothalamic disorder.

In the fourth ventricle, ependymoma is the commonest tumour. In addition to raised intracranial pressure it may cause vomiting or vertigo as an isolated feature.

The key investigations in these cases are computerised axial tomography and ventriculography with air or Myodil. Benign tumours may be excised but removal of a large mass may be technically difficult.

PINEAL AND PARAPINEAL TUMOURS

Tumours in this area are seen particularly in adolescents and young adults. They include teratoma, pinealoma, glioma, and a cyst. The characteristic features are paresis of vertical gaze, pupils resembling the Argyll Robertson pupil, hydrocephalus and hypothalamic disorder. The presence of a mass is confirmed by computerised axial tomography or ventriculography. Access to this area for biopsy is difficult, and excision of the tumour is likely to increase the neurological deficit. It is now thought preferable to relieve the hydrocephalus with a shunt from the ventricle to the cistern and follow this with radiotherapy. The pinealoma is highly sensitive to radiotherapy.

Shunting Procedures. Measures designed to divert the flow of cerebrospinal fluid may give relief when the ventricular system is obstructed or there is failure of absorption. This may be done as a preliminary to dealing with the cause of the obstruction by surgery or radiotherapy.

The earliest of these procedures was third ventriculostomy as when a communication was established between the third ventricle and chiasmal cistern. This is satisfactory as a short-term therapy but the stoma may close and the application is limited.

A plastic tube may be used to drain fluid from the lateral ventricle to the cisterna magnum (Torkildsen). When this is not feasible, a tube with a valve (Spitz–Holter or Pudenz–Heyer) may be used to drain fluid to the atrium, pleura, or peritoneal cavity. There is some risk of infection, and the tube may have to be replaced.

TUMOURS INVOLVING THE VISUAL PATHWAY

In any patient with progressive visual failure that is not attributable to glaucoma or other disease of the eye, the possibility of compression of the visual pathway demands consideration. The optic nerve may be compressed by a meningioma arising in the sphenoidal ridge or olfactory groove. A glioma of the optic nerve is rare, and usually seen in children. These tumours are likely to cause proptosis. At the chiasma, compression may be due to pituitary tumour, meningioma, cranio-pharyngioma, or, occasionally, aneurysm. Tumours that involve the posterior visual pathway include glioma, meningioma, and arteriovenous malformations.

Glioma of the Optic Nerve and Chiasma. A rare tumour that is most often seen in children and particularly in association with multiple neurofibromatosis. It may present with visual loss, proptosis, pain, or as an amblyopic eye. Tumour tissue may be visible at the optic disc and the optic foramen is often enlarged. The hypothalamus may be involved.

Radical excision is seldom possible, but some of these tumours evolve only very slowly over many years. Surgery may be needed to control proptosis. The place of radiotherapy is controversial, but shrinkage of the mass is reported in some cases.

Pituitary Tumour. The most common pituitary tumour is the chromophobe adenoma which erodes the sella, compresses the visual pathway, and may cause hypopituitarism. The eosinophil adenoma causes acromegaly. The basophil adenoma associated with Cushing's syndrome rarely causes compression. Pituitary apoplexy may be the presenting feature (page 128).

Preliminary tests of endocrine function are desirable. These include blood and urinary cortisol, growth hormone, and serum T4. Even when they are normal, the period of operation should be covered with hydrocortisone (50 mg six-hourly).

Surgical removal is usually the treatment of choice. If the tumour is large or the visual pathway is involved a transcranial (frontal) approach is usually preferred. Small tumours may be removed by the transnasal route and sometimes yttrium 99 is implanted to ablate the gland. Alternatively, and particularly when there is no compression of the visual pathway, radiotherapy may be used.

In patients with gigantism or acromegaly, surgical removal of the tumour is advised if there is chiasmal compression. Often the sella is not much enlarged and its appearance in a lateral radiograph is not a good guide to the hormone activity of the mass. The expectation of life in patients with acromegaly is significantly reduced, and heart disease is the main cause of death. The level of growth hormone in the blood is a useful guide, and when it is raised, even in the absence of features of chiasmal compression, radiotherapy, excision, or ablation of the tumour mass should be considered.

Postoperative irradiation of the sella is usually advised. In this way any fragment of tumour remaining may be destroyed, and the recurrence rate is reduced. Transient diabetes insipidus is usual after hypophysectomy and it may persist. This can be controlled with pitressin tannate by daily injection or dearginine vasopressin inhalation (DDAVP). When the gland has been removed, maintenance therapy with 25 to 50 mg of cortisone acetate and 0·1 to 0·3 mg thyroxine daily will be needed for life.

Craniopharyngioma. This tumour arises from a persistent embryonal remnant. It may evolve at any time of life and is sometimes recognised in old age. The usual presenting features are headache, visual failure, endocrine disorder, and loss of memory. The intracranial pressure may be raised. Endocrine features may include hypogonadism, arrest of growth, diabetes insipidus, and hypopituitarism. The tumour mass is often adjacent to the tuber cinerium. It may invade the third ventricle or, occasionally, the sella. Small areas of calcification may be seen above the sella in a lateral radiograph of the skull.

Surgical treatment is difficult. It is seldom possible to excise the tumour because it is closely adherent to other structures. Relief of hydrocephalus may be achieved by means of a shunt. Visual failure may necessitate decompression of the chiasma, and the mass is often cystic. It is important that the endocrine state is controlled, and replacement therapy with corticosteroid, thyroxine, and antidiuretic hormone may be needed. There may be a place for growth hormone in children. The main danger of operation is the risk of injury to the hypothalamus and hypophysis. If excision is impossible, radiotherapy should be considered. Control of the cyst to prevent accumulation of fluid may be attempted using ^{32}P or ^{198}Au injected through a burr hole and under radiographic control. There is a risk of leakage of the isotope and its spread beyond the cyst.

In conclusion, the endocrine management is important, and radical excision is sometimes possible, particularly in children. In the adult, control of the cysts may give prolonged relief.

RADIOTHERAPY

The place of radiotherapy in the treatment of brain tumours is difficult to assess. This is partly because the exact extent of the tumour is often not known, and there is a tendency on the part of some surgeons to refer patients whose tumour could not be excised completely for radiotherapy. The value of radiotherapy seems to be established in medulloblastoma of the cerebellum, brain stem glioma, and as a means of reducing the risk of recurrence of pituitary adenoma. In craniopharyngioma, chiasmal glioma, cerebral hemisphere glioma, and inoperable meningioma, its value is more doubtful. Dosage must be controlled as there is a risk of late radiation necrosis. This usually occurs from 12 to 18 months after the treatment and the clinical features may suggest (and be wrongly interpreted as) a recurrence of the tumour.

Chemotherapy and isotope therapy for cerebral tumour cannot yet be said to have passed the experimental stage. The management of meningeal reticulosis and leukaemia is discussed on page 225.

THE INOPERABLE TUMOUR

Every neurologist has witnessed the circumstances of the patient with minimal symptoms whose investigation at an early stage indicates a glioma, large or small. It poses a serious dilemma in management. If a drill biopsy is done the patient may be made worse. Exploration by open craniotomy to obtain a biopsy is less likely to increase in the neurological deficit. Sometimes the histology is inconclusive. In the face of subsequent clinical deterioration it is clear to all concerned that the disease is progressive. When the diagnosis is known and the patient relatively fit, it is difficult to decide how much he should be told. Only a few people seem to be able to live with the knowledge that they have an inoperable brain tumour, and preserve equanimity. Experience in dealing with such patients suggests that it is not always in the best interest of the patient to push the diagnostic investigation to the extreme at an early stage, but no general rule can be laid down.

When it is clear that an inoperable tumour is present, what can be done? In some cases simple analgesics may give relief from headache. Anticonvulsant drugs usually control epilepsy. Headache due to raised intracranial pressure can be controlled for a variable time (sometimes many months) with dexamethasone. The initial dose should be small, e.g. 4 mg daily, but may have to be increased in steps up to 20 mg daily. If it is stopped there is likely to be a rapid deterioration. In the absence of evidence of raised intracranial pressure or progressive focal neurological deficit, it is probably wiser to withhold corticosteroid therapy.

By these methods it is often possible to maintain the patient in good general condition until the terminal phase of the illness. At that point nursing care becomes the major consideration.

When the diagnosis is clear, it is important that the situation is explained to a responsible relative. If this is not done, a worsening of the condition is likely to lead to loss of confidence in the doctor. It is one of the most difficult arts of medical practice to decide how much to tell the patient at any given stage. It is perhaps well for the practitioner to reflect that he is not the only source of information, but this should not lead him to the simple expedient of telling every patient the full details of his illness, even when the patient seems to be demanding it.

15

Developmental Disorders

Malformations of the brain or spinal cord are found in about six per thousand births and account for a third of all malformations. A high proportion of these children are stillborn or die within the first month of life.

Several factors have contributed to bring these patients into prominence in recent years. The sex may be determined and chromosomal abnormalities may be detected by examination of the cells in amniotic fluid. Maternal rubella and the administration of thalidomide during early pregnancy have emerged as causes of malformation. Success in the control of infection and surgical measures such as shunts to relieve hydrocephalus have resulted in survival of handicapped infants. A generation of disabled children has stimulated thought about the ethics of treatment that allows survival in the presence of gross mental or physical disability.

Examination by fetoscopy of the child in utero after the 18th week of pregnancy can be used to confirm the presence of anencephaly or meningomyelocele. Study of the amniotic fluid after the 13th week may reveal chromosomal abnormality in mongolism. Biochemical investigation of enzymes can be used to recognise some metabolic disorders. Phenylketonuria can be diagnosed at birth by examination of blood or urine, and then controlled by diet (page 246).

Multiple anomalies may be present and it is common for hydrocephalus to be associated with meningomyelocele.

ABNORMALITIES OF THE CRANIUM

Enlargement of head may be due to hydrocephalus from any cause and this must be distinguished from macrocephaly. With encephalocele and craniostenosis the skull is abnormal in shape. Microcephaly is sometimes associated with epilepsy and may be due to intrauterine infection with cytomegalic virus, rubella, or toxoplasma Gondii.

Macrocephaly refers merely to the upper range of normal skull size. It is distinguished from hydrocephalus by the normal rate of growth, normal size of the ventricles, and absence of other clinical features.

An *encephalocele* develops in the midline and may arise at any point between the nasion and occiput. It is often associated with a bone defect and appears in the early months of life. Occipital encephalocele may continue into the cerebellar area or be associated with the Chiari malformation. Air ventriculography is necessary to define the abnormality. The treatment is surgical; it consists of excision of the sac, and repair of the skull defect with a bone graft. There is a high incidence of associated handicap.

Craniostenosis is due to premature fusion of the bones of the skull and may result in compression of the cranial contents. The effect may be asymmetrical or distort the shape as in turricephaly. Craniostenosis of the vault can be relieved by surgical excision of strips of bone but the base cannot be dealt with in this way.

Hydrocephalus. The term implies an excess of fluid within the cranium in relation to the volume of the brain. It is commonly associated with obstruction to the flow of cerebrospinal fluid but investigation is necessary to establish the cause. Only a few cases are diagnosed at birth. The condition commonly shows itself several months later with enlargement of the head, bulging fontanelle, separation of sutures, and depression of the eyes. Papilloedema is not a feature.

The differential diagnosis must consider macrocephaly (when cranial enlargement is the only feature), subdural effusions which may be related to trauma (often associated with retinal haemorrhage), and tumour. Cerebral tumour is suggested by the presence of papilloedema, or a later onset. Good quality plain radiographs are essential. The investigation is mainly directed to the ventricular system and an air ventriculogram is usually done. The computerised axial tomogram and isotope encephalogram are sometimes helpful. Hydrocephalus and subdural effusions may complicate meningitis in infancy.

When diagnosis is established, careful assessment is needed. There may be associated lesions such as aqueduct stenosis, tumour, arachnoid cyst, porencephaly, subdural effusion, or myelocele, which require surgical treatment. If these are excluded the question to be answered is whether the condition is progressive. If it is mild or not progressive a period of observation may be the best course. The majority deteriorate if not treated and later show mental retardation, spasticity, optic atrophy, and a high incidence of epilepsy. Occasionally, aqueduct stenosis presents in the adult and the clinical features suggest a posterior fossa tumour.

In most cases the treatment consists of introducing a shunt to allow ventricular drainage. When the aqueduct is obstructed an opening may be made in the third ventricle (ventriculostomy) but it may not be sufficient. The use of a shunt requires insertion of a plastic tube fitted with a valve so that there is flow in only one direction. One end is placed in the lateral ventricle and the tube is subcutaneous throughout most of its course to the cardiac atrium or peritoneal cavity. The valves in common use are the Holter and Pudenz-Heyer.

The early results are good and in some cases, even if the tube becomes occluded, an important phase of development may have passed and equilibrium be re-established. Rapid release of high intraventricular pressure may provoke a subdural haematoma. The catheter may be occluded in the heart by thrombus. Pulmonary embolism may lead to pulmonary hypertension. Infection in the tube is sometimes difficult to control and it may have to be replaced. Growth of the child may result in retraction of the catheter tip.

The Dandy-Walker syndrome is found in early uterine life when the foramina which drain the fourth ventricle are occluded. The fourth ventricle expands and compresses the brain stem and cerebellum. Development of the cerebellum is arrested. The clinical features are those of hydrocephalus associated with cerebellar disorder; the diagnosis is made by air ventriculography. Relief can be obtained by ventriculocisternotomy (Torkildsen) or some other shunting procedure.

ABNORMALITIES NEAR THE FORAMEN MAGNUM

An abnormal contour of the occiput and neck may be seen clinically, and often the neck is short. Plain radiographs will clarify the situation.

Basilar Invagination. In this condition the cervical spine is placed high in relation to the skull base because the ring of the foramen magnum is invaginated. Confirmation is obtained from radiographs, and several diagnostic criteria have been described. McGregor's line extends from the dorsal margin of the hard palate to the caudal point of the occipital curve as seen in a lateral radiograph. If the odontoid is more than 9 mm above this line the base is invaginated (Bull). Antero-posterior tomograms help to define the invagination. When there is evidence of compression of the lower brain stem or spinal cord, surgical removal of the lower part of the occipital bone and posterior lip of the foramen magnum may give relief.

The *Klippel-Feil syndrome* is an association of short neck, low hair line, and restriction of neck movements. Radiographs show fusion of some or all of the cervical vertebral bodies, the number of cervical vertebrae may be reduced, and other anomalies may be associated. Turner's syndrome is sometimes present. Treatment is not required for Klippel-Feil syndrome but it should direct attention to other abnormalities.

Arnold-Chiari Malformation. The essential feature is the displacement of the hind brain into the cervical canal. It is classically associated with meningomyelocele but may occur in isolation or with hydrocephalus. The displacement may not give rise to neurological disorder and skeletal abnormalities may be associated. There may be pressure effects at the foramen magnum and obliteration of space by arachnoidal adhesion. The clinical features may suggest syringomyelia, medullary or cord compression, a cerebellar disorder, or raised intracranial pressure. Sometimes the lower cranial nerves are involved. Trauma, even of a minor kind, may aggravate the condition.

Investigation is by plain radiographs in the first instance. Contrast methods with air or Myodil may also be required.

Surgical treatment may be needed to relieve compression but the procedure adopted will be determined by the particular problem. Decompression of the foramen magnum posteriorly is the usual method.

ABNORMALITIES OF THE SPINAL CORD

Meningomyelocele is often associated with hydrocephalus. The less severe meningocele and spina bifida occulta are important. Diastematomyelia usually presents in childhood and syringomyelia in early adult life. Stenosis of the spinal canal and kyphoscoliosis may be found in isolation or be associated with other developmental abnormalities.

Spinal Dysraphism. Of the children with spina bifida cystica (2/1000 births) about a fifth are stillborn. The survivors can be subdivided into a minority with simple meningocele which respond well to treatment and a majority with meningomyelocele, often associated with hydrocephalus, which carry a poor prognosis.

Simple Meningocele. A midline defect of fusion is most common in the lumbar region. The membrane does not bulge at birth but may protrude later. Rupture of the sac leads to meningitis. Hydrocephalus develops in some but may stabilise without treatment. There is no abnormality of the spinal cord. Early surgical closure of the defect is satisfactory and a high proportion of these children develop normally.

Meningomyelocele. In addition to the failure of membrane fusion the cyst contains neural tissue and is most often located in the thoraco-lumbar region. It commonly involves several segments, the spinal cord is abnormal, and there is a high incidence of associated hydrocephalus. If the superficial defect is closed the infant may be protected from the risk of meningitis but only a very small proportion develop normally. The majority have weakness of the lower limbs, disturbance of the sphincters, and mental retardation.

Spina Bifida Occulta and its Assessment. While meningocele and meningomyelocele can often be recognised by inspection and palpation of the spine at birth, less marked abnormalities may come to light at a later stage of development. The diagnosis of these is important because growth may lead to traction effects and disability which can sometimes be prevented by surgical treatment.

The cardinal features are skin abnormalities, spinal curvature, abnormal lower limbs, and incontinence of urine. The skin lesion may be a dimple, a tuft of hair, or a sinus. This may be an isolated feature but should lead to a search for the other abnormalities and neurological signs of disorder of the lower limbs. Plain radiographs may show spina bifida. When there is evidence that the disturbance is more than superficial, myelography will be required. This will define the outline of the spinal cord and any associated features. At operation the findings may include a low conus medullaris, diastematomyelia, intradural lipoma, fibrous bands, or a cyst.

The aim of surgery in these cases is to prevent deterioration in the lower limbs or loss of control of the sphincters. The area is explored and it may be possible to divide fibrous bands and restore the normal mobility.

Diastematomyelia. This term implies a longitudinal division of the cord. There may be duplication (diplomyelia) or a cleft. The defect is commonest in the lumbar region but may extend into the thoracic region. The disorder usually presents with weakness in the legs or features of cord or root involvement. Sensory loss is often found and the sphincters may be involved.

Plain radiographs may reveal a bony spur in the lumbar or lower thoracic region and myelography is needed to define the anatomy of the spinal cord. Surgical treatment should be carried out early because the cord is commonly tethered to the bony spur or one of the lower vertebrae and becomes stretched as growth continues. The spur is excised together with the septum in order to release the cord.

Ethical Considerations. The simplicity of closure of a spinal defect has resulted in survival of a number of disabled children who would otherwise have died from infection. Some of these have severe and multiple disabilities which condemn them to a vegetative existence. This has given rise to doubts about the wisdom of an unselective policy of surgical closure of all spinal defects. Selection presents both practical and ethical difficulty because the operation to close the defect is often straightforward and best done on the first day of life. The decision whether to proceed has therefore to be made at once.

If it is accepted that some severely disabled children should not have the defect closed the question arises, what are the factors which indicate a poor prognosis? An assessment of all disabilities is the first step. Those found to have severe flaccid paraplegia, kyphosis, severe clinical hydrocephalus, gross heart disease, or cerebral birth injury have a high incidence of subsequent morbidity and a high mortality. Often there is a large thoraco-lumbar myelocele in these cases.

Lorber suggests that if one or more of these major factors are present the operation should be discussed with the parents and the prognosis explained. A decision not to proceed with the operation may then be reached.

Syringomyelia. Investigation and surgical treatment of this condition has been stimulated by the hypothesis proposed by Gardner to explain its development. Gardner postulates that the initial disturbance is obstruction to the flow of spinal fluid at the medial or lateral foramina of the fourth ventricle. Over a period of years this results in a disturbance of the dynamics of fluid flow and a damming back of fluid with consequent distension of the central canal of the spinal cord. While this may explain most cases it should be pointed out that in others there is no communication between the syrinx and the ventricular system. A cavity in the cord may also arise in association with arachnoiditis, a tumour, local trauma, and as a late complication of traumatic paraplegia.

In the typical case there is scoliosis, weakness and wasting of the small muscles of the hands, absence of tendon jerks in the upper limbs, increased jerks in the lower limbs, extensor plantar responses and dissociated sensory loss over the upper limbs and trunk. Other features include Horner's syndrome, nystagmus, and neuropathic joints of the upper limb. The gross and long established clinical state is irreversible.

Surgical treatment should be considered if a communicating syrinx is present. Investigation is by myelography with air or Myodil and this must be performed with the patient supine to show prolapse of the cerebellum. If cerebellar ectopia is found, sub-occipital decompression with cervical laminectomy is indicated. At operation the anatomy of the cerebellum is restored as far as possible, obstruction to the flow of cerebrospinal fluid is relieved, and ventricular drainage ensured. This may improve function but also offers the best hope of arresting progression. The presence of adhesions may cause difficulty, and attempts at mobilisation may then give rise to haemorrhage or injury to the medulla.

Stenosis of the Spinal Canal. The capacity of the spinal canal shows considerable variation. If it is narrow, the mobility of the cord will be constrained and degenerative changes or minor prolapse of the intervertebral discs may lead to cord compression. A narrow canal may be part of a generalised skeletal disorder such as achondroplasia but it is also found as an isolated feature.

The treatment of spinal compression in achondroplasia may be unsatisfactory because the canal is narrow throughout its length. Compression is most marked in the dorsal region. Lumbar canal stenosis is discussed on page 190.

Scoliosis. In the neonatal period this condition is likely to be associated with gross disorder of the nervous system. When it develops later in childhood or adolescence it is most commonly idiopathic but a few of the cases are secondary to neurological disease.

If the scoliosis is mild when first seen, frequent observation is required to detect any progression. If there should be the spine is immobilised, using a Milwaukee brace and plaster. When the condition has stabilised wedge resection may be performed.

Pes Cavus. Pes cavus is an exaggeration of the arch of the foot which may be associated with claw toes or a club foot. It may be congenital or acquired. In a small proportion of cases it is associated with hereditary neuropathy, Friedreich's disease, or myelodysplasia.

Thalidomide and Malformation. The drug thalidomide which was in general use as an hypnotic in the 1950s and early 1960s was found to cause fetal abnormality when given to women in early pregnancy. The main disorder was a failure of development of the limb (phocomelia) but in some cases there were more widespread defects. Some or all of the limbs might be absent. This problem has stimulated work in the design of mechanical limbs which has reached a high degree of sophistication.

CEREBRAL PALSY

This term is applied to non-progressive brain disorders present at birth or recognised in early childhood and manifest as a motor disability. The group is not of common aetiology. Birth injury and many other factors such as prematurity, prolonged labour, asphyxia, and convulsions may contribute. The condition is seldom hereditary.

The group is usually classified on the basis of the dominant motor features as diplegic, hemiplegic, monoplegic, ataxic, choreiform or athetoid. There may be associated disorders of the special senses or brain function.

Some of the features may not be apparent until it is noted that the milestones of development are delayed.

Cerebral palsy is seen in about 2 per thousand of live births. The majority develop spastic limbs, and about a quarter are subject to epileptic attacks. About half have some ocular disorder but less than 10 per cent are blind. A fifth are deaf and more than a fifth show mental retardation. More than half are able to lead an independent existence and be employed.

Assessment. The first stage in management is assessment of the physical and mental handicap. This is best done by a team accustomed to working with these problems. It will include the family doctor, paediatrician, orthopaedic surgeon, otologist, ophthalmologist, neurologist, child psychiatrist, health visitor, and physiotherapist. At a later stage the speech therapist may participate.

The aim of treatment is to promote normal physical and mental development within the limits of the disability, by advice to the parents, and supportive therapy.

Counselling Parents. Any approach to the treatment of a child must include discussion with the parents and explanation of the needs so that full co-operation is obtained.

When an abnormality is revealed in the child the emotional impact on the parents is often marked. They require support in coming to terms with the problem and this is best provided by the family doctor helped by the health visitor and others. It is often found that explanations given at an early stage are not grasped because of the emotional disturbance, and have to be repeated. Explanation must be linked with support and appropriate reassurance. The degree of reassurance must be determined by the clinical situation and its likely course. Prediction of the outcome becomes more exact as progress is watched. There is no place for blind reassurance, on the one hand, or unrelieved gloom, on the other. A realistic and honest appraisal, erring perhaps a little on the side of optimism, is the only one that is likely to carry conviction over a period of years.

The reaction of the parents to unpalatable news will be determined by their own culture, character, insight, and education. A common initial response is to reject the child, and this may be coupled with feelings of guilt and despair. The situation may be aggravated by misunderstandings and sometimes conflicting opinions. It is always wise to find out from the parents what they have already been told so that a clear picture emerges. It is important that the report of what has been said is passed on to the family doctor and others who are concerned in the management of the child.

Management in Infancy and the Early Years. The emphasis is on training and physiotherapy. When there are epileptic attacks appropriate and regular anticonvulsant therapy is started and modified according to progress. The mother will need advice about holding the child and methods of promoting satisfactory posture. A suitable chair has a long back and sides with a slight backward and downward tilt of the seat. Training in feeding, toilet, and dressing requires perseverance and often has to be prolonged. As growth continues, physiotherapy is increasingly directed to the activities of the child and the control of posture. Orthopaedic advice may be needed about the use of splints, braces and suitable shoes or boots in conjunction with physiotherapy. Speech therapy is valuable in assessment and in ensuring maximal function. The severely deaf child will need special training for speech and education. It is important to appreciate that intelligence may be normal when there is spasticity, deafness, or a speech disorder.

School Life. When the age of five is reached a more comprehensive assessment will be possible and plans for education are made. Some children with cerebral palsy can attend an ordinary school but those with mental retardation or severe disability require a special school.

Attendance at school may be associated with particular difficulties for these children. Often they have been relatively isolated at home and lack contact with other children. The parents tend to be over-protective and problems of adaptation to the school routine may arise. Intelligence becomes a major factor in determining the limits of achievement. Every effort is made to ensure as normal a school life as possible.

As school life continues it becomes possible to arrive at a realistic approach to future life and employment. It is important that plans made should not be over-ambitious because this leads to much frustration.

Adolescence. The progress made at this stage will depend not only on intelligence, disability and the previous training, but on acquired skills and the capacity for independent activity. The school environment provides protection and support that may not be available later. Social adaptability is therefore an important consideration.

Further education and employment may be arranged through the Youth Employment Service and Disablement Resettlement Services.

Adult Life. The less severely handicapped may adapt to a normal way of life. There is a tendency to frustration and isolation. Some become dependent on a relative and lead a narrow existence which is abruptly changed when illness or death removes the support. The more severely disabled live in Cheshire Homes or other institutions, but attempts should always be made to keep them in the community. Community living may be supported by Day Care Centres and other provisions for group activities.

16

Spinal Cord Disorders

Acute spinal cord trauma and the investigation and management of the various causes of spinal cord compression are the main subject of this chapter. Multiple sclerosis, which frequently enters in the differential diagnosis of a spinal cord lesion, is dealt with in Chapter 11.

PHYSICAL SIGNS

An acute myelopathy may cause flaccid weakness with absent tendon reflexes and indeterminate plantar responses. There is sensory loss below the lesion. Subsequent improvement of cord function is associated with a spastic weakness, increased tendon reflexes and extensor plantar responses. The abdominal reflexes are absent when damage is in the mid-dorsal region or above. In incomplete lesions the sensory loss may be dissociated or light touch and position sense may be predominantly involved. In chronic spinal cord disease there is no flaccid phase. Radicular pain is common with spinal cord tumours, or cervical spondylosis and local pain over affected vertebrae may be present with extradural neoplasm. If there is retention of urine, the need for surgical relief of spinal compression is urgent.

DIFFERENTIAL DIAGNOSIS

In acute spinal trauma the commonest cause of spinal cord damage is fracture dislocation of the spine. Acute compression of the cord may be due to vertebral collapse from metastases, myeloma, or reticulosis. Acute cervical cord contusion or haematomyelia may result from acute hyperextension or flexion injury to the spine in the presence of cervical spondylosis and a narrow spinal canal.

Myelography is required where any possibility of cord compression exists. Apart from identifying spinal cord tumours and spondylytic myelopathy, a negative myelogram may assist in the diagnosis of transverse myelitis and multiple sclerosis.

It is most important to give urgent consideration to the possibility of spinal cord compression in any patient with progressive loss of power and sensation in the lower limbs. A delay in referral to a suitable centre often results in irreversible paraplegia.

In practice, conditions such as motor neurone disease and the myelopathy of vitamin B12 deficiency seldom present a diagnostic problem. Spinal syphilis is now very rare. It may be confused with cervical spondylosis or a cord tumour but examination of the CSF and appropriate serology will confirm the diagnosis.

MYELOGRAPHY

The radiological investigation of spinal cord lesions using the subarachnoid injection of positive contrast media is an essential diagnostic technique. Myodil (ethyliodophenyl-undecanoate) is widely used. Myelography with air or water soluble medium is an alternative technique. The lumbar route for myelography is preferred unless it is necessary to show the upper level of a spinal block or where more than one lesion is suspected and a spinal block has been demonstrated; one may then introduce Myodil by cisternal puncture. In cervical examinations 9 ml of Myodil is recommended for use and 12 ml for dorsal lesions.

The complications of myelography include root pain radiating down the legs, headache, infection, and an aseptic meningitis. Occasionally, the latter is severe enough to justify the use of corticosteroids. Policy about whether to remove Myodil or not is in doubt. We recommend removal of as much Myodil as possible although it must be accepted that this is not always technically easy. Reactions to Myodil are unpredictable but are sufficiently frequent to justify a positive approach to removing the substance.

The types of abnormality seen at myelography assist in distinguishing extradural, intradural, and intramedullary compression of the spinal cord. An extradural block usually has a serrated margin. Intradural tumours usually show a rounded filling defect and the spinal cord may be seen to be displaced. In intramedullary tumours the spinal cord is expanded and the Myodil flows round it. The expansion covers several segments.

In cervical spondylosis lateral protrusions cause failure of root sleeve filling and a lateral defect in the Myodil column. Posterior filling defects cause a hold-up in the Myodil flow which is most marked in the extended neck position when the posterior longitudinal ligament buckles.

Myelography is normally performed in the prone and supine positions. Supine myelography is particularly important in investigating syringomyelia when herniated cerebellar tonsils may be outlined (page 163).

ACUTE SPINAL CORD TRAUMA

In civilian life the majority of spinal cord injuries are the result of direct trauma to the vertebral column, in contrast to the high number of penetrating injuries in war. Injuries to the lower thoracic and lumbar spine are commoner than cervical and upper dorsal trauma. In cervical injuries, violent movement of the neck is important. C5-6 and C6-7 are the most affected levels. Flexion and rotational injury to the dorsal spine or pressure transmitted through the feet is responsible for many dorsal injuries. Fracture dislocation may still be evident at the time of examination or the subluxation may have reduced spontaneously. In the view of many, total loss of spinal cord function below the level of injury for 48 hours means there will be no functional recovery. There are rare exceptions to this rule.

Immediate Management. When moving the patient, the body should be moved as one, with gentle traction on the cervical spine in a neutral or slightly extended position. Traction should be applied to the feet as well. There should be cushioning under the dorsal spine and behind the knees. At the site, an assessment should be made of the possibility of other injuries and the degree of paralysis.

At the hospital, X-rays of the whole spine may reveal the majority of fractures and dislocations. The neurological and general status will be reviewed. High cervical lesions may require respirator care while the assessment is completed. A spinal injuries unit should be contacted immediately and transfer arranged whenever possible. No decisions about operation or major treatment measures should be undertaken without this contact.

Management of the Bone Injury. After 48 hours there is little likelihood of operation being of any value except in particular circumstances. An important but rare exception is an acute soft cervical disc protrusion.

Myelography will reveal a soft tissue swelling in front of the spinal cord. Operative removal produces good results. Decompressive laminectomy for a swollen cord is of no value. In the cervical region, most subluxations are reduced by traction on the skull using up to 20 lb (9 kg). In the dorsal region the position of the spine is best maintained by cushioning. Fracture dislocations in the thoraco-lumbar region involving the conus and cauda equina may benefit from open reduction because there may be some benefit to the cauda equina. Surgery is indicated if there are obvious intraspinous spicules of bone which may be relevant to the injury and where a partial cord lesion is worsening.

General Management. Most aspects of this are dealt with elsewhere. The skin is protected by frequent turning from the supine to the lateral, back to the supine, and then to the contralateral position. The turn should be made at least every two hours.

Bladder function is managed by intermittent catheterisation. Once urine flow is established this needs to be carried out three times daily. The work done by Guttmann suggests that catheterisation has a lower infection rate than other methods. The object is to establish reflex micturition.

The bowels are best aided by the addition of lubricants and fibre to the diet. In the early stage of traumatic paraplegia absorption is impaired and the serum protein may fall. A high protein appetising diet helps to overcome this and the low morale that may prevent adequate food intake.

Spasticity is helped by making sure the patient is free from infection and pressure sores. Diazepam, baclofen and dantrolene may help. The positioning of the limbs has a bearing on whether paraplegia in flexion or extension develops. There is no firm evidence that the severity of the cord lesion is relevant. The legs should therefore be placed in an extended position with slight flexion at the knees. Paraplegia in flexion should be avoided.

Rehabilitation. Eventual rehabilitation is greatly helped by the facilities of the paraplegic centre and the opportunity to be with similar patients. Determination and general morale are most important.

Patients with dorsal lesions are able to learn transfer activities and move on to walking with the aid of crutches and full length leg braces. Upper limb muscles need to be developed, in particular latissimus dorsi. However, the amount of energy expended in trying to walk increases with the height of the lesion, and most patients with mid or upper dorsal damage find walking too exhausting.

Transfer from bed to chair is achieved by placing the chair with brakes on beside the bed and grasping the arm of the chair with the appropriate limb. The other arm is then used to push the body upwards so that it can be swung into the chair. The legs are then positioned manually. Some people prefer to use hoists. Transfer to a bath is helped by grab rails and may be made straight from a chair or from an intermediate seat.

In cervical lesions, damage at C4 and above is not normally compatible with life. Some movement is possible with C5 lesions and below this activity increases. The use of gadgets that can be slipped round the fingers may aid in feeding and communication.

Sensitive electronic equipment activated by microswitches (possum) enables the quadriplegic patient to turn lights on and off, turn pages, use television and carry out a wide variety of functions. Blowing or sucking on a mouthpiece is sufficient to activate the equipment, and the life of a quadriplegic patient can be transformed.

CERVICAL AND DORSAL DISC PROTRUSIONS

Lateral cervical and lumbar disc protrusions are covered in Chapter 17. Acute central soft cervical disc protrusions are rare in contrast to those in the lumbar region. Trauma is a relevant factor in many cases. The presenting feature is usually that of a rapidly progressive spastic paraparesis often associated with motor or sensory signs in the arms. The diagnosis can only be made by myelography when a soft tissue mass is seen lying in front of the spinal cord at the level of a disc space. Urgent operative treatment is required. This may be achieved by posterior approach but the technical difficulties of extracting disc material from in front of the cord are considerable. An anterior approach is the preferable route and, provided the cord is not damaged, the operative results are excellent.

Dorsal disc protrusion is a rare cause of significant neurological disability. Lateral protrusions cause thoracic root pain but this is not an indication for radical intervention. Such pain frequently settles down with rest. A central protrusion will cause spinal cord compression and is difficult to distinguish from other causes of cord pathology in this region. Plain X-rays of the dorsal spine may reveal a calcified disc—an important sign. Trauma is a factor in most cases. The operative treatment is difficult. The narrow diameter of the dorsal canal combined with the anterior position of the protrusion make operation a hazardous procedure. There may be postoperative paraplegia, and even in expert hands the morbidity is considerable.

CERVICAL SPONDYLOSIS

Spinal cord compression due to cervical spondylosis is related to a congenitally narrow spinal canal. In the presence of a wide canal, compression is unusual except in the presence of gross osteophytic formation. There may be a mixed cord and root compression syndrome, and root pain and sensory disturbance in the arms may result from root compression or cord involvement. The most important cord feature is a spastic paraparesis. The evolution of the spastic weakness may be slow with periods of static disability. The cord syndrome due to cervical spondylosis is often regarded as self limiting but there may be progression over several years. The problem in the management of cervical spondylosis is in part due to lack of agreement on the indications for operation and the type of procedure to be employed. There is still a need for critical evaluation of operative results. Trials of operative treatment have proved difficult to establish.

Investigation and Diagnosis. The diagnosis may be suspected in someone with a spastic paraplegia where there is a history of recurrent neck or root pain and when cervical movements are limited.

Plain radiology of the cervical spine should include anteroposterior, oblique and lateral films. Lateral views should be obtained in a neutral position, and flexion and extension to assess stability.

Myelography is required to assess the levels involved and to exclude the possibility of a tumour which may be the cause of compression even when cervical spondylosis has been demonstrated on plain radiology; 9 ml of Myodil are used. A hold-up in the extended neck position is usually present if the spondylosis is significant. Caution must be exercised in attributing a paraparesis to spondylosis in the presence of minor myelographic findings. Failure of root sleeve filling should be noted and assessed in relation to root signs in the arms.

Treatment. Conservative management is indicated when the patient is elderly and when general medical considerations make operation unwise. In the presence of a mild myelopathy a period of observation is justified, especially if the myelographic findings are unconvincing.

The conservative management of root pain is rest in bed with support for the neck for a period of at least two weeks. A short period of bed rest may also improve the myelopathy. Cervical traction with skull calipers relieves many cases of acute root pain.

The use of a collar will reduce neck movements and any instability that exists. The most important points about choosing the correct collar are that it should fit properly, restrict neck movement, and be comfortable.

Surgical treatment is largely a choice between an anterior and posterior approach. An anterior fusion with removal of degenerate disc material is a useful operation when the disease is localised to one or two levels at the most. There is little postoperative pain. It is unwise to perform the operation in the presence of a long narrow spinal canal and when multiple levels are involved. Laminectomy at several levels and often from C2-C7 will relieve compression. It is unwise to combine this with any attempts to remove osteophytes although foraminotomy at one or two levels may be done at the same time. Some regard foraminotomy as important in maintaining cord blood supply via the radicular arteries. Following a widespread laminectomy it is advisable for the patient to wear a collar for up to six months. This reduces instability, which may be responsible for late deterioration following surgery.

The results of surgical operation for myelopathy are difficult to evaluate. Improvement may be expected in about 50 per cent of cases. Further deterioration should be prevented. The results are less good when multiple levels are involved. Operation should not be delayed until an advanced stage of disability has been reached as the results are poor.

INTRASPINAL TUMOURS AND CYSTS

Spinal compression due to tumours and cysts produces varied physical signs in relation to the site and nature of the compressing cause. Intraspinal tumours may be extradural, intradural, or intramedullary. Extradural compression may result from the spread of a vertebral lesion. Cervical tumours produce upper and lower motor neurone signs in the arms according to the site. A high cervical tumour may produce false localisation in the form of wasting of the small muscles of the hand. It appears that the grey matter in the spinal cord is more susceptible to anoxia than fibre tracts. The motor pathways are particularly prone to the effects of ischaemia and compression. Although it may be possible to ascertain the likely nature of cord compression preoperatively, it usually requires operative intervention to be certain.

The most important causes of extradural compression are metastatic carcinoma, reticulosis, and myeloma. Tuberculosis is an important cause in certain parts of the world, as is hydatid disease. Intradural tumours are usually benign and the neurofibroma and meningioma are the most important. The neurofibroma is the commonest benign spinal cord tumour.

It is most frequent in the cervical and lumbar regions. The meningioma is the common benign tumour in the dorsal region and is more frequent in women. Intramedullary tumours are usually gliomas. The ependymoma is the commonest spinal glioma followed by the astrocytoma. Intramedullary gliomas may be cystic.

EXTRADURAL COMPRESSION

Extradural cord compression is normally due to some form of malignant neoplasm. Infection such as tuberculosis or an extradural abscess are important non-neoplastic causes. Pain is a common presenting symptom. Both must be recognised early to avoid serious cord damage. Extraspinal tuberculosis and radiological evidence of erosion of vertebral bodies adjacent to a disc space are helpful signs. A paravertebral shadow may be seen. In extradural abscess, severe local pain and a very high ESR are usual. A local source of infection may be present. Extradural abscess is discussed on page 226 and Pott's paraplegia on page 224. Pain may be localised over a vertebral body involved by malignant disease. Once cord compression is evident progression is rapid. Plain radiology of the whole spine may reveal multiple bony lesions and a collapsed vertebrae at the appropriate level. It is vital to arrive at a precise pathological diagnosis before a final decision can be made about detailed management.

Metastatic Carcinoma. This is now a common cause of extradural cord compression. The dorsal cord is more often involved than the cervical cord. Carcinoma of the lung, breast, and prostate represent three of the more important sites, but compression may be caused by neoplasms from a wide variety of origins. Spinal cord compression may be the presenting manifestation of malignancy. This is more likely with carcinoma of the lung and prostate.

Although the prognosis may be poor, histological verification of the diagnosis should be obtained whenever possible. A clinical examination and screening procedure may not reveal an obvious primary. Chest examination and an examination of the breasts with mammography may be needed. A search for prostatic carcinoma may be made with a rectal examination and estimation of the acid phosphatase. If there is suspicion of an alimentary or renal lesion then barium studies and an intravenous pyelogram should be performed. If there is a bone lesion at the spinal level, myelography is unnecessary as one can assume the clinical localisation has been accurate.

Laminectomy and biopsy should be performed when the primary is unknown and there is no lymph node to take for histological diagnosis. When the diagnosis is known there is often ambivalence about the desirability and value of laminectomy and removal of what tissue is possible. On the whole, the prognosis following operation is not good and worthwhile recovery is seldom seen. On the other hand, most surgeons have experience of a gratifying response in individual cases, particularly in instances of carcinoma of the breast and prostate. It is reasonable to recommend laminectomy when the cord lesion is incomplete and, in particular, when sphincter function is preserved. If the patient is in a poor clinical state and the cord lesion is complete, operation is not indicated.

Laminectomy may be followed by radiotherapy in suitable cases. Radiotherapy is not a satisfactory substitute for laminectomy when there is marked cord compression. Hormone therapy has a place in the management of carcinoma of the breast and prostate but the local problem should be dealt with surgically. The place of cytotoxic drugs in the management of metastatic carcinoma is still under evaluation but there is no firm evidence that it is of value in spinal cord compression due to metastatic carcinoma.

Reticulosis and Myeloma. Extradural cord compression due to Hodgkin's disease usually indicates widespread disease. The diagnosis may normally be made by biopsy of material other than the cord lesion. There may be cord compression early in the disease or as a complication after therapy has started. Although modern combined chemotherapy has revolutionised the prognosis of advanced Hodgkin's disease, laminectomy should be performed in the presence of cord compression. This applies to other forms of reticulosis in adults. Cytotoxic drugs alone or combined with local radiotherapy should be given after laminectomy.

Myeloma may be solitary or disseminated. The diagnosis of myelomatosis made by the demonstration of an abnormal serum protein band, Bence-Jones proteinuria, and a positive bone marrow biopsy. In solitary myeloma, histological diagnosis has to be made at operation. Following decompression, radiotherapy should be given at the appropriate level, and treatment with cytotoxic drugs should be used in multiple myeloma.

INTRADURAL COMPRESSION

The meningioma and neurofibroma are the two most important intradural neoplasms. Both are benign. On rare occasions the meningioma may be extradural and, occasionally, intramedullary. The neurofibroma may arise near to the intervertebral foramen. In this case a dumb-bell tumour may form and present in the thorax or neck rather than as a cause of cord compression. The diagnosis of intradural cord compression depends on myelopathy. There are no characteristic physical signs. Root pain is more likely with a neurofibroma. There may be widening of the spinal canal or enlargement of intervertebral foramina with a neurofibroma. A widened canal is seen less frequently with a meningioma.

Neurofibroma. This tumour is commoner in the cervical and lumbar regions. In the latter it causes cauda equina compression. As the tumour arises from a nerve root, there will be pain of radicular type. Most neurofibromata arise from posterior nerve roots. In the early stages there may be an ipsilateral pyramidal weakness combined with contralateral dissociated anaesthesia.

After myelography, removal is effected by laminectomy. It is usual to carry out a complete removal. The relevant posterior nerve root has to be sacrificed. If the spinal cord has not been compressed for a long time, excellent recovery over the next four months can be expected. After prolonged compression, improvement will be slow but the cord has remarkable powers of recovery.

Meningioma. The tumour is most common in the dorsal region and has no particular clinical characteristics. Operation is often more difficult than with a neurofibroma. The tumour may be highly vascular and the origin from the dura may be wide. Delivery of the tumour may have to be piecemeal. Recurrence is more likely and particularly when the tumour is anteriorly placed and the dural attachment is inaccessible without risk to the cord. On the whole, the outlook is similar to the neurofibroma. Postoperative radiotherapy is not required.

INTRAMEDULLARY NEOPLASMS AND CYSTS

Gliomas. Most intramedullary neoplasms are gliomas. The ependymoma is the commonest but many of them cause cauda equina compression rather than cord compression. The neoplasm may be expansile or infiltrating. Characteristically dissociated sensory loss on both sides occurs in the region of the tumour. Anterior horn cell involvement may be a feature and produce progressive scoliosis when the tumour is in the dorsal region. Usually there is sacral sparing, even when there is widespread sensory loss.

At operation, the cord may be expanded over a few segments or there may be a fusiform swelling over a wide area. The swollen cord may be solid or soft indicating an underlying cyst containing yellow fluid with a high protein content. This will distinguish it from the cystic cavity of syringomyelia.

A widespread laminectomy should be performed. The ependymoma and astrocytoma form the commonest types of glial tumour. Whether the tumour can be removed depends on its invasive properties. A solid astrocytoma may be removed if there is a clear plane of cleavage. A spinal glioma extending over many segments is extremely difficult to extirpate and radical surgery is likely to lead to damage to the descending and ascending pathways. If removal is impossible a biopsy may be taken and any cyst drained. Approximately 13 per cent of spinal cord gliomas may be totally removed, and most of these are ependymomas. An ependymoma may be shelled out through a posterior midline incision. The dura should be left open and radiotherapy given. Disability depends on whether the tumour has been successfully removed and the degree of spinal cord damage. Many spinal cord gliomas are slow growing and patients may live for many years.

INTRASPINAL CYSTS

These cysts may be extradural, intradural or intramedullary. Developmental spinal arachnoid cysts are rare causes of cord compression. They are usually dorsal. Dermoid cysts are relatively common. They are most frequent in the lumbar region. The diagnosis is made at operation and the cyst may be successfully excised. Enterogenous cysts lined by columnar or cuboidal epithelium are often associated with widespread defects of the neural arch. They may be successfully removed although there may be difficulty if the cyst is anterior to the cord or intramedullary. Endothelial cysts are usually relatively simple to excise. In certain areas hydatid cysts are common. They are frequently extradural and multiple. Although there may be excellent remission, recurrent compression is common and the ultimate prognosis unfavourable.

VASCULAR TUMOURS AND MALFORMATIONS

A haemangioma of the vertebral body may be associated with extradural compression. The radiological appearance of the vertebra is characteristic. There is well-marked vertical trabeculation of bone against a background of diminished bone density. The height of the vertebra is usually diminished. The best treatment is radiotherapy without operation. Laminectomy may be associated with massive haemorrhage, and the results of irradiation are good. The haemangioblastoma is similar to the tumour found in the posterior fossa. The tumour may grow in a nerve root or on the surface of the cord. It may also be partially embedded in the cord. The successful removal of such tumours is possible if they lie outside the cord. Radiotherapy is of value postoperatively.

Vascular malformations of the cord are complex. The development of angiographic techniques have allowed visualisation of the individual radicular feeding vessels. The treatment of choice is to excise the angioma completely. The malformation must lie outside the cord with clearly defined feeding vessels and the blood supply to the cord assured. Such circumstances prevail in approximately 30 per cent of malformations. It is claimed that up to 70 per cent of patients may be improved by the ligation of feeding vessels. This is an area of neurosurgery where those with a special interest in the subject have accumulated experience that justifies referral of such patients to appropriate centres.

17

Disorders of the Cranial Nerves and Peripheral Nervous System

Under this heading we are concerned with the cranial nerves, nerve supply to muscle, and sensory connections with the spinal cord. The anterior horn cell, which is the cell body (perikaryon) of the motor nerve, lies within the spinal cord and gives rise to the anterior nerve root which merges with the sensory fibres and continues as peripheral nerve. The sensory neurone begins at a sensory receptor and, after running in the peripheral nerve, separates to form the posterior root which carries the ganglion and enters the spinal cord. It is clear, therefore, that motor and sensory fibres lie adjacent throughout most of their course in the peripheral nervous system.

An important difference between the axons of peripheral and central neurones is the capacity of the former for regeneration, provided the cell body is intact.

Trauma is a major factor in peripheral nerve disease. Seddon recognises three degrees of injury: neurotmesis, axontmesis, and neuropraxia. From the pathological standpoint, disease may affect the cell body, axon, or myelin sheath (segmental demyelination). Dying back neuropathy begins at the periphery. These pathological groups are not mutually exclusive and often coexist in the same nerve.

Clinical Features. Motor and sensory features are often combined. There may be weakness, muscle wasting, fasciculation, and loss of tendon jerks. Paraesthesiae with sensory loss is common. Cranial nerves may be involved. Respiratory paralysis threatens survival. Sphincter functions are often preserved, but sometimes lost. Autonomic disturbance may cause impotence, postural hypotension, loss of sweating, and trophic changes in the skin.

Electrical Studies. Electromyography is helpful in distinguishing peripheral neuropathy from myasthenia and myopathy. Neuropathy causes a reduction in the interference pattern due to loss of motor units, and signs of denervation. Denervation is shown by the presence of fasciculation (spontaneous discharge of a motor unit), positive sharp waves, and fibrillation (spontaneous contraction of single muscle fibres). In myasthenia, there is progressive decrement in amplitude of the units evoked by electrical stimulation. In myopathy, the interference pattern is retained until an advanced stage is reached, the amplitude, and the mean potential duration is reduced, but there is little or no spontaneous activity.

Nerve conduction velocity can be measured in accessible peripheral nerves by recording the response to electrical stimulation. It is possible by this means to obtain the velocity in the fastest conducting fibres only. Motor velocity is obtained by supramaximal stimulation at two points along the nerve, with recording of the muscle potential and latency. The difference in latency between the two points gives the time for the impulse to pass from one to the other, and when the distance is measured the velocity can be calculated. Sensory nerve velocity is more difficult to measure because nerve potentials are small. The nerve is stimulated with skin electrodes, and the potential recorded from surface electrodes or a needle placed alongside the nerve. The latency for supramaximal stimulation is obtained. It is important that the limb is kept warm and the temperature controlled. Normal velocity is of the order of 50 to 70 m/sec. A reduction in conduction velocity of about a third is commonly associated with segmental demyelination. Marked slowing, i.e. to 15 m/sec, is found when there is widespread destruction of large fibres.

Nerve conduction may be normal when there is a lesion of the root; the H reflex may then show a delay. If, for example, the common peroneal nerve is stimulated and the response recorded with skin electrodes over the calf, two distinct potentials will be seen. The first potential is due to direct stimulation of the motor nerve. The second potential is due to weak stimuli passing to the spinal cord and returning to the muscle. This may show increased latency in root disease.

Terminal latency measurements obtained by supramaximal stimulation of the motor nerve close to the muscle are useful in the diagnosis of entrapment such as carpal tunnel syndrome and other peripheral neuropathies.

Nerve Biopsy. The method is limited in application and can be conveniently used only for the sural nerve and superficial branch of the radial nerve. Excision of the sural nerve leaves the patient with numbness around the fifth toe, but in the setting of a peripheral neuropathy this is of little moment. It is not possible to measure conduction velocity in the intact sural nerve.

The procedure for sural nerve biopsy is carried out under local anaesthesia. The nerve lies in the midline of the calf posteriorly and is conveniently located over the lower third of the leg. A longitudinal incision is made through skin and fascia. About 10 cm of nerve is removed, care being taken to avoid injury. The specimen is fixed. Fixation in formalin-mercuric chloride-acetic acid (Susa) is suitable for conventional and silver stains. Chromic acid and osmium (Flemming) is appropriate for myelin stains. Gluteraldehyde or formol-calcium is suitable for teasing fibres and electron microscopy (Bradley).

CRANIAL NERVES

Ophthalmoplegia. Ophthalmoplegia may arise from disease of the brain stem; compression or other disorder of the oculomotor, trochlear, and abducent nerves, myasthenia, or myopathy. If the brain stem is involved there are likely to be other neurological signs. Compression of the nerves will cause progressive effects. In myasthenia the weakness fluctuates and is reversed with edrophonium chloride (Chapter 18).

Exophthalmos with Ophthalmoplegia. The diagnostic possibilities will include thyroid disease, cavernous sinus thrombosis, carotico-cavernous fistula, orbital tumour, orbital pseudotumour, and mucocele of the ethmoid sinus. Papilloedema may be associated. The first three are likely to produce bilateral effects, but hyperthyroidism is also a common cause of unilateral exophthalmos.

Proptosis with oedema of the conjunctiva, lid retraction, and lid lag suggest thyroid eye disease. This may be preceded or followed by clinical hyperthyroidism or latent hyperthyroidism revealed by chemical tests. The titre of thyroid antibodies in the blood is often raised. The treatment of thyroid exophthalmos is often difficult. If the patient is hyperthyroid, this is controlled with radioactive iodine or antithyroid drugs. In mild cases repeated observation is important and the exophthalmos may progress when the patient is euthyroid. A lateral tarsorrhaphy may be needed to protect the cornea. In more severe cases prednisolone 140 mg daily is given to relieve oedema. If control is not obtained within a few days or visual failure develops, orbital decompression may be needed. Decompression may be followed by local radiotherapy.

Cavernous sinus thrombosis usually follows infection of the face or septicaemia. There is headache with orbital oedema, ophthalmoplegia, and sometimes papilloedema. The eye involvement may be unilateral at first and there may be visual failure. Orbital phlebography will confirm the diagnosis. The infection must be treated vigorously with antibiotics and anticoagulant therapy is then given. The condition is now uncommon. Full recovery is possible.

In patients with carotico-cavernous fistula, there is intense venous congestion, exophthalmos (sometimes pulsatile), cranial bruit, ophthalmoplegia, and papilloedema. The diagnosis is confirmed by carotid arteriography, which shows the communication, and the contrast medium may pass from the artery to the jugular vein without perfusing the brain. Spontaneous closure sometimes happens but surgical treatment is usually needed. Simple ligation of the carotid artery proximal to the fistula may aggravate the situation by causing blood to drain from the hemisphere into the fistula. It is necessary, therefore, to ligate the artery both proximal and distal to the fistula or, ideally, to close the fistula, but this is a difficult procedure.

An orbital tumour will produce pain, proptosis, and visual failure. Plain radiographs may show erosion of the sphenoidal ridge, which suggests a meningioma. If metastatic tumour is excluded as far as possible by examination of the breasts, palpation for enlarged lymph glands, and chest radiograph, further special radiography may be needed. The most useful techniques are the computerised axial tomogram, orbital phlebogram, and arteriogram of the orbit. These investigations will usually demonstrate a mass, and may indicate its nature. Surgical treatment is then required and may be followed by radiotherapy.

Ophthalmoplegia without Exophthalmos. This may be part of a generalised neuropathy as in the Guillain-Barré syndrome, the prognosis for recovery then being good. It also occurs in association with migraine (Chapter 6). Abducent nerve palsy, unilateral or bilateral, is seen in patients with raised intracranial pressure, and is then of no value in localising the cause. It clears when the pressure is relieved. Isolated abducent palsy is not uncommon in patients over 50 years of age with or without diabetes mellitus. Most cases resolve in about three months, and it is usually regarded as vascular in origin.

An isolated third nerve palsy is more likely to indicate a compressive lesion, but can happen with diabetes mellitus. Posterior communicating artery aneurysm may present in this way, and usually there is pain as well. When there is oculomotor palsy after head injury it suggests that haematoma has formed and, in the patient with raised intracranial pressure, it may indicate herniation of the tentorium. Treatment is then directed to the cause. Direct compression of the nerve may be due to tumour—commonly a meningioma.

The *Tolosa-Hunt syndrome* (painful ophthalmoplegia) is rare and may be related to collagen vascular disease. In a typical case there is pain, ophthalmoplegia, a raised blood sedimentation rate, and positive antinuclear factor in the blood. Arteriography may show narrowing of the carotid syphon, and orbital phlebography may show occlusion of the superior orbital vein. The condition responds to corticosteroid therapy. Prednisolone 60 mg daily may be given improvement developing in a few days. After ten days the dose can be reduced gradually, and the therapy stopped after a month. There is, sometimes, a relapse. The condition must be distinguished from ophthalmoplegic migraine which may be recurrent, and the high erythrocyte sedimentation rate, positive antinuclear factor, and other serological tests for collagen disease are useful in differentiation.

The *orbital pseudotumour syndrome* shows links with Tolosa-Hunt syndrome, and endocrine exophthalmos. The term covers a group of patients with pain, exophthalmos, trigeminal neuropathy, and sometimes a slightly elevated protein level in the spinal fluid. There may be visual failure. Corticosteroid therapy such as prednisolone 20 to 50 mg daily may give relief and is then continued for several weeks and gradually withdrawn.

Trigeminal Neuropathy. Trigeminal neuralgia is considered in Chapter 6. Pain and sensory loss over the face may be due to compression of the nerve or its central connections. It may be a feature of brain-stem tumour, infarction, or demyelination. A trigeminal neuroma is uncommon, but may cause pain and progressive sensory loss over the face. The sensory loss associated with multiple sclerosis often clears in a few weeks.

Nasopharyngeal carcinoma may present with facial pain and numbness. This tumour is common in the Far East, but rare in Europe. It may cause nasal discharge, nasal obstruction, or epistaxis, and the diagnosis of a nasopharyngeal tumour is then likely to be considered. Plain radiographs may show a soft tissue mass and bone erosion. Basal radiographs of the skull are helpful and may reveal erosion around the foramen ovale and foramen rotundum. In patients who present with cranial nerve palsy, the trigeminal, abducent, and hypoglossal nerves are often affected, but any nerve may be involved. Enlarged lymph glands may be palpable in the neck. The diagnosis is confirmed by biopsy of a gland or of the mass in the nasopharynx. Nasopharyngeal examination may be difficult and a general anaesthetic is often required. The presence of cranial nerve palsies indicates spread beyond the confines of the nasopharynx. The treatment is radiotherapy, but results are poor.

Trigeminal neuropathy is also seen in progressive systemic sclerosis and other collagen diseases. It evolves rapidly and may be bilateral. Pain is sometimes prominent. The numbness persists and is not much influenced by corticosteroids or other treatment.

Trigeminal neuropathy is also reported as a benign condition that clears in a few weeks.

Protection of the eye is important when corneal sensation is impaired. This may be achieved with spectacles fitted with a shield over the lateral part of the orbit. When this is insufficient, a tarsorrhaphy is performed.

Facial Palsy. An isolated lower motor neurone facial palsy in an adult may follow trauma, herpes zoster, brain-stem disease, or neuropathy, but the commonest variety is Bell's palsy.

The cause of Bell's palsy is unknown. Some cases are associated with hyperacusis or loss of taste over the anterior part of the tongue on the same side. Either of these features indicates that the lesion in the facial nerve is proximal. Most cases make a clinical recovery, but a few improve slowly over a period of two years and about 15 per cent have some permanent residual weakness.

Since the majority recover without treatment, there is a need to identify those with a poor prognosis. Most palsies that are incomplete recover fully. Electrical tests are of no value in the first few days. In the second week, electromyography may show fibrillation waves that indicate denervation. Stimulation of the nerve at the angle of the jaw causes the orbicularis oris to contract, and this can be recorded. Absence of this response in the second week suggests a poor prognosis, and a normal or increased latency is usually a favourable sign. The problem here is that the electrical signs are too late a feature to help in deciding early treatment.

Surgical decompression of the stylomastoid foramen and nerve canal has been widely practised, but is of no proven value. Electrical stimulation is not effective in treatment. Splinting of the face may improve the appearance.

Patients with complete Bell's palsy seen within a week of the onset should be given prednisolone 80 mg daily for five days, provided there is no contra-indication. Those with severe residual weakness persisting for two years from the onset may be helped by hypoglossal-facial anastomosis.

When herpes zoster is the cause of a facial palsy, pain is prominent and the incidence of residual weakness is about 50 per cent.

Crocodile tears provoked by eating (gusto-lachrimatory reflex) may develop after facial palsy. Relief can be obtained by interruption of the glossopharyngeal nerve at the jugular foramen, or close to the ear drum. This is first done with local anaesthetic and, if effective, can be followed by nerve section. If this fails, relief may be obtained by blocking the sphenopalatine ganglion, and if tears are controlled, the ganglion can be destroyed by injecting absolute alcohol.

Gustatory Sweating. This may arise as a consequence of abnormal reinnervation after surgical operation on the parotid or submandibular gland, or thoracic inlet, and sometimes as a complication of diabetic autonomic neuropathy. It may respond to propantheline, and surgical treatment is better avoided.

Multiple Cranial Nerve Palsies (cranial polyneuritis). This may be part of a generalised neuropathy in the Guillain-Barré syndrome. Metastatic tumour is a common cause, and the primary lesion may be in the nasopharynx. A few cases are due to sarcoid and this may also cause an isolated cranial nerve palsy (most commonly the facial nerve). The diagnosis of sarcoid depends on biopsy and histology of a gland or other tissue. Some cases respond to corticosteroid therapy. The initial dose of prednisolone is usually about 60 mg daily, and if a response is obtained, the therapy is gradually reduced to the minimum required to control the condition.

Syphilis is a rare cause and multiple cranial nerve palsies may occur in any type of granulomatous meningitis.

SPINAL NERVE ROOTS

Radiculopathy may be multiple or confined to a single root. Pain and weakness are often prominent, but when the sensory root is involved there may be paraesthesiae and sensory loss. As examples, acute polyneuropathy and the syndrome of root compression will be described.

Acute Polyradiculopathy (Guillain-Barré syndrome). The neurological illness is often preceded by an acute infection, and the condition is generally regarded as an allergic neuropathy. Neural involvement begins with paraesthesiae, pain, and weakness. The tendon jerks are lost at an early stage. The condition may evolve in the course of a few hours, and sometimes leads to quadriplegia. It may take a fortnight to reach peak severity, or occasionally longer. Bulbar paralysis and respiratory failure may supervene. The spinal fluid may be normal at first, but usually there is a rise in protein without any increase in the cell count. Respiratory failure or secondary infection may lead to death but if controlled most patients make a full recovery.

Management in the acute stage requires all facilities for intensive care. Adequate fluid intake and nutrition may need a gastric tube if there is bulbar paralysis. Respiration must be carefully observed, and assistance with it may be needed for several weeks (Chapter 1). To protect the skin it is essential to turn the patient frequently. Passive movement of the limbs to prevent contracture at first, may be replaced by active exercises later. Back splints to support the ankles and wrists are useful. Simple aids that support a book and turn the pages, and other mechanical devices, give the patient some independence. Treatment may have to be continued for weeks or months, but in many cases improvement begins in the second or third month, and may continue over several years. Sometimes there is a relapse.

The place of corticosteroid therapy is not yet clear. Moderate doses such as 100 mg of prednisolone daily have little effect in most cases. A small proportion do respond, and some are corticosteroid-dependent. The responsive group can only be identified by trial of corticosteroids, and this is advised in severe cases. If there is no response within a fortnight, the drug can be withdrawn.

Recently, there have been reports of high dosage corticosteroid therapy, methyl prednisolone being given intravenously up to 1 g daily, and continued for a week. The value of this has yet to be assessed.

Antibiotics have little place except when there is secondary infection. When the acute stage has passed, a prolonged period of rehabilitation may be needed.

Acute Radiculopathy due to Intervertebral Disc Prolapse. The dominant feature is pain, and there may be weakness and sensory loss. There is disc prolapse, commonly, in the cervical or lumbosacral spine.

In the cervical region it may be provoked by whiplash injury or come on spontaneously. There is pain in the neck and arm. Often the triceps jerk is lost. Relief is obtained by immobilisation, using a collar. If pain persists, neck traction may be used (Chapter 2). In the early stage there may be confusion with herpes zoster, tumour, or compression due to other causes. In patients with acute radiculopathy due to disc prolapse there is no indication for urgent surgical treatment.

Sciatic pain is most often due to lumbar disc prolapse. It may be provoked by lifting a heavy object. There is often a history of low back pain which spreads down the back of the thigh and may reach the toes. Commonly, there is painful limitation of straight leg raising and loss of the ankle jerk. There may be foot drop and other motor deficit with sensory loss as well. In many of these cases the pain settles in a few weeks, but when focal signs are present myelography may be indicated to define the site of prolapse. We prefer to restrict myelography to those in whom surgical treatment is contemplated. When there are focal signs they may be taken as indicating the site of prolapse. Pain responds to rest in bed and analgesics. In acute sciatic pain the use of prednisolone 30 to 60 mg daily may give relief and can then be reduced gradually over a period of two or three weeks.

In the early stages, bed rest on a firm mattress is advised and essential if the pain is severe. Many cases settle with this alone in the course of a week or two. A disc protrusion in the dorsal region is unusual, and when seen appears mainly in those doing heavy manual work. It may cause intercostal pain. Sciatic pain or persistent backache in a child is unlikely to be due to disc prolapse, and if it persists myelography should be considered, even in the absence of localising signs, when it may reveal a meningioma or neurofibroma.

In milder cases it seems that time is more significant than immobility. Surgical treatment is seldom urgent except when the bladder is involved. Disc protrusion in the lower part of the spinal canal may cause a cauda equina syndrome. This is discussed separately.

Brachial Plexus Neuropathy (neuralgic amyotrophy). The condition is characterised by the development of pain around the neck and shoulder with weakness and wasting that may be very marked. It can sometimes be seen to follow about ten days after an injection of foreign protein, as in vaccination or immunisation. It may be unilateral, and is sometimes confined to a single nerve such as the phrenic, or the nerve to serratus anterior. Recovery is usual, but may take many months. A striking feature is the restoration of muscle bulk and function with recovery.

The disorder is regarded as allergic in origin, but evidence of this is not found in all cases. It may be precipitated by trauma, and is commoner in males.

Treatment is helped by making a firm diagnosis in the first instance, and avoiding traumatic investigation. Analgesics are needed to relieve pain. Corticosteroid therapy has not been found effective. Gentle physiotherapy to preserve joint mobility is useful in the early stages, and more active exercises later. Surgical exploration should be avoided.

Trauma to the Brachial Plexus. This is a complication of traction on the upper limb or penetrating injuries. The distribution of weakness and sensory loss will indicate the roots involved. Interruption of the posterior root will cause sensory loss and, if peripheral to the ganglion, there is loss of nerve conduction and the cold vasodilatation response. If the lesion is supraganglionic these responses may be preserved, but the prognosis is poor. Cervical myelography may show enlargement of root sheath spaces and formation of meningoceles as a consequence of traction. Surgical exploration is of limited value, particularly in supraclavicular lesions; it is discussed in detail in Seddon's monograph. In general, brachial plexus lesions due to trauma have a poor prognosis for recovery.

Thoracic Outlet Syndrome. Paraesthesiae and numbness of the fingers and upper limbs have in the past been too frequently attributed to compression of nerves passing over the first rib by the scaleneus anterior muscle, or a prominent cervical rib. In most instances this is not the cause, and the origin of the pain is more likely to be found in cervical spondylosis or carpal tunnel syndrome. The possibility of a malignant tumour involving the nerve roots must be considered, and careful palpation of the neck, supra-clavicular region and axillae is needed. Horner's syndrome may be found on the same side. Bronchial carcinoma arising at the apex of the lung is an important cause (Pancoast tumour). There are a few well-documented cases in which compression at the thoracic outlet does cause numbness, pain, and paraesthesiae over the ulnar aspect of the hand and forearm with wasting of the hand muscles. There may be an elongated transverse process of the C7 vertebra of rudimentary cervical ribs. At operation, a fibrous band that extends from these structures to the first rib is found. Division of the fibrous band relieves pain and paraesthesiae.

Spinal Arachnoiditis. This uncommon condition can only be diagnosed at operation or by myelography. It may be associated with spondylosis, tumour, chronic inflammation, such as tuberculosis and cryptococcal infection, sarcoid, radiation, and trauma, and in the past has been attributed to syphilis. Metastatic tumour, injection of toxic substances such as phenol and radio-opaque media into the spinal theca, Beçhets syndrome and collagen disease produce similar effects. The main symptom is pain, and there may be neural or spinal deficit from local traction. This condition is commoner in the Far East. In acute cases provoked by contrast media, corticosteroid therapy may control the condition.

Cauda Equina Syndrome. The spinal cord ends at the upper border of the L2 vertebral body but the canal continues to S2. The nerves to lower lumbar and sacral segments pass close together in this region, and may be compressed. The clinical features are pain, disorder of bladder and bowel, numbness over the saddle area, and root involvement which commonly causes wasting of the gluteal and thigh muscles and loss of knee and ankle jerks.

The sudden onset of these features must be regarded as a surgical emergency, particularly when sphincter function is impaired. Common causes include intervertebral disc prolapse, stenosis of the spinal canal, and tumour either primary or secondary, injury, and bone disease. Radiographs of the lower spine and chest may show bone destruction or tumour, but myelography will usually be needed. It is important that relief of urinary retention by catheter should not lead to delay in dealing with the underlying cause before irreversible effects are produced. The reduction of pain in this situation is not always a favourable feature as it may indicate that a root that at first was irritated has been compressed so that function is lost.

A chronic cauda equina syndrome may be due to a tumour such as a neurofibroma or intervertebral disc protrusion, and is sometimes aggravated by trauma. Pain is usual, and the onset of bladder disturbance makes investigation urgent. Some patients have stenosis of the spinal canal, and even a minor disc protrusion may then cause compression. This group of patients may present with pain in the back and thighs which is provoked by exercise and relieved by rest (neurogenic claudication). Surgical decompression gives relief.

Occasionally, a cauda equina syndrome is produced by invasive tumour outside the spinal canal, such as myosarcoma.

PERIPHERAL NERVES

The clinical subdivisions between radiculopathy and neuropathy are arbitrary and reflect the emphasis of pathological effect, for there is often overlap. Polyneuropathy and mononeuropathy will be described separately, but the later stage of multiple mononeuropathy resembles polyneuropathy.

Polyneuropathy. Many causes have been described, and a substantial group remains in which no cause can be established, particularly among the elderly. In some systemic disorders such as diabetes mellitus, signs of peripheral neuropathy are commonly present and nerve conduction slowed even in the absence of symptoms. It is important to look for predisposing causes. Investigation begins with examination of the urine and a chest radiograph. Spinal fluid examination often shows a raised protein level. The serum vitamin B12 level, glucose tolerance, blood urea, liver function tests, blood count, plasma proteins and electrophoresis should be done. Tests for antinuclear factor, latex test, and sheep cell antibody may reveal collagen disease.

Studies of nerve conduction velocity and measurement of terminal latency are useful in making the distinction between demyelination and axonal neuropathy. Demyelination causes a reduction in velocity. In axonal neuropathy the evoked potential is reduced in amplitude but velocity may be normal. Terminal latency is increased in 'dying back' neuropathies.

The general management is to ensure adequate fluid intake and nutrition (which may demand a lot of supportive help if the patient is paralysed), and protection of the skin by frequent turning. Pain may require analgesics, and sensitive hands may be relieved by using cotton gloves. Vitamin therapy is commonly administered, but is of little value.

Diabetes Mellitus. The neuropathy may be the presenting feature and mononeuropathy is common. Much dispute has centred on the question whether control of the metabolic disorder influences the neuropathy. The neuropathy may be predominantly sensory and associated with ulceration of the feet. Neuropathy is more common in the severe and long-standing diabetic, but is also found with the latent disease. It is often assumed that control of the diabetes will lead to improvement, but this cannot always be shown. When pain is prominent, the use of insulin may give relief even when not strictly necessary to control blood sugar. It must be used cautiously because hypoglycaemia can cause a neuropathy.

In the neuropathy that has been called diabetic amyotrophy there is pain and weakness of thigh muscles and loss of the knee jerks. It is frequently asymmetrical. Control of the blood glucose leads to improvement.

Autonomic effects can often be demonstrated in diabetes mellitus, but the common symptoms are impotence and diarrhoea. Bradycardia may be a prominent feature.

Renal Disease. Neuropathy is common in patients with renal failure. Some relief may follow dialysis, but the neuropathy may be aggravated or provoked at first. Successful renal transplantation leads to improvement over a period of months (*see also* page 239).

Hepatic Disease. Clinical neuropathy is rare. Sometimes in the alcoholic, both liver cirrhosis and neuropathy are present. Liver failure more commonly affects the central nervous system (*see* Chapter 18). In primary biliary cirrhosis, xanthomatous deposits in the nerves may cause sensory neuropathy.

Porphyria (*see* Chapter 20). Acute porphyria should be considered in any obscure neuropathy. There may be abdominal pain and mental confusion. The urine contains porphobilinogen, and develops a port wine colour on standing. The most important aspect of management is the avoidance of drugs that provoke it, such as barbiturates, sulphonamides, and oestrogens.

Vitamin Deficiency (*see also* Chapter 20). Neuropathy is a feature of beri beri, but the only common cause in Western Europe is vitamin B12 deficiency. It is usually part of the pernicious anaemia syndrome. It begins with paraesthesiae and numbness followed by weakness, and commonly progresses over the course of a few weeks. The diagnosis is confirmed by finding a blood level below 100 ng/litre, and it is rare to meet with neurological features when it is higher than this. Hydroxycyanocobalamin is given by daily intramuscular injection at first (1 mg) and then reduced in frequency. It must be continued for life, usually at intervals of a month. The symptoms do not always clear completely, and residual signs are common.

Other vitamin deficiencies may cause a similar neurological picture. Thiamine deficiency is common in the Far East where rice forms the staple diet, and it is found in alcoholics and patients with gastrointestinal disease. It may also cause the Wernicke-Korsakow syndrome. The pyruvate mechanism is impaired. The metabolic effects can be corrected by giving thiamine 100 mg daily i.m. for a week. The daily requirement is about 1 mg. Nicotinic acid deficiency causes pellagra which responds to nicotinamide 50 mg daily i.m. Pyridoxine deficiency may be associated and will be mentioned in relation to isoniazid.

When there is malnutrition, alcoholism, or gastrointestinal disease, a course of injections of vitamins B and C (Parentrovite) should be given daily for ten days. Oral supplements of vitamins are seldom indicated when the diet is satisfactory.

Poisons and Drugs (*see also* Chapter 20). Many metals cause neuropathy, including arsenic, thallium, and lead. Some are used in treatment, such as gold and antimony. Alcohol is an important factor, but the mechanism is nutritional deprivation, and particularly vitamin B1 deficiency.

Some drugs cause neuropathy, a possibility that should always be considered when seeking the cause. Isoniazid is more likely to do so in those in whom it is metabolised slowly, and it is rare when the dose is 300 mg daily or less. It can be prevented by giving pyridoxine 10 mg daily. Nitrofurantoin, used in the treatment of bladder infection, may cause neuropathy if its excretion is delayed by renal failure, and this may be permanent. Chloroquine is an occasional cause, the neuropathy improving when the drug is withdrawn. Thalidomide also caused an irreversible neuropathy affecting the lower limbs and was predominantly sensory. Phenytoin may cause a chronic neuropathy with loss of tendon jerks.

Carcinomatous Neuropathy. Carcinoma may involve peripheral nerve or roots directly, but there is also a systemised neuropathy in patients with carcinoma (particularly of bronchial origin), reticulosis, and myelomatosis. The malignant disease may be latent and only revealed after months or even as long as two years. Remission of the neuropathy sometimes happens in untreated cases. When the tumour is removed or treated by other methods, the neuropathy is likely to persist. There is no satisfactory treatment.

Hereditary Neuropathy. The commonest is Charcot-Marie-Tooth disease, which is quite often autosomal dominant and usually evolves slowly through adult life. The signs of peripheral neuropathy may be combined with claw hand, pes cavus, and thickening of peripheral nerve. Nerve conduction velocity may be very slow but in some varieties is normal.

Some other hereditary neuropathies with sensory involvement lead to ulceration of the feet, and there may be necrosis of the bones of the foot. These trophic changes can be delayed by care of the skin and provision of suitable shoes.

In Refsum's syndrome, neuropathy is combined with ataxia and pigmentary degeneration of the retina. The serum phytanic acid is high, and may be reduced by a diet low in chlorophyll which may arrest the disease.

Collagen Disease. Neuropathy is a feature of polyarteritis nodosa but it is also seen in rheumatoid disease and systemic lupus erythematosus. It may be localised to isolated nerves, and histological examination may show arteritis of the small vessels. Mononeuropathy may evolve into multiple mononeuropathy, and in some cases the neuropathy is symmetrical and generalised. In the acute case with active disease and a high erythrocyte sedimentation rate there may be a good clinical response to corticosteroid therapy. The initial dose may be prednisolone 60 mg daily, but if there is no response it should be increased until the sedimentation rate is controlled. The dose can then be reduced gradually. Not all cases respond, and in chronic cases it may be better to avoid steroid therapy.

MONONEUROPATHY

Mononeuropathy is most commonly seen as a consequence of trauma or entrapment. It is found in leprosy (page 229), diabetes mellitus, and the collagen diseases.

Trauma and Entrapment Neuropathy. Pressure effects may be occupational, as in the motor palsy of the deep branch of the ulnar nerve in those using screwdrivers and similar tools.

Neuropathy of the Lateral Cutaneous Nerve of the Thigh (meralgia paraesthetica). In this condition the patient is aware of numbness and tingling sensations with pain over the lateral aspect of the thigh. Sensory loss may be demonstrated over the affected area. The condition may be bilateral, and is most often seen in middle-aged obese males. It is due to traction or compression of the nerve when it penetrates the fascia or the inguinal ligament. Explanation and reassurance are usually sufficient. In persistent cases section of the nerve can be performed, but the residual paraesthesiae may give trouble and it is better avoided.

Carpal Tunnel Syndrome. This is commoner in women and may be bilateral. In bilateral cases the presence of a systemic disorder such as rheumatoid disease, hypothyroidism, acromegaly, or myeloma should be considered. Unilateral cases may be related to local fracture or injury, but in most there seems to be an occupational factor. The complaint is pain, numbness, and tingling in the index and middle fingers. Characteristically, the paraesthesiae wake the patient at night, and are relieved by holding the hand high out of bed. The pain may spread to the forearm and arm.

Examination may show sensory loss of median nerve distribution. The thenar eminence may show wasting, and weakness of abduction and other movements of the thumb may be demonstrated. Pressure over the carpal tunnel may provoke the symptoms.

Measurement of the terminal motor latency of median nerve conduction, which assesses transmission across the carpal tunnel, exceeds 3 ms in most cases, and may be prolonged to 10 ms.

The definitive treatment is surgical decompression of the carpal tunnel.

It requires full exposure of the flexor retinaculum and complete division of it. Operation relieves the sensory features, but muscle-wasting may persist. In pregnancy it can be relieved by injection of hydrocortisone into the carpal tunnel, this also being a useful diagnostic test in doubtful cases.

Injection of the carpal tunnel is best carried out without local anaesthetic under sterile conditions. A short needle (2 cm) of fine bore with a small syringe containing 25 mg of hydrocortisone in 1 ml of oil solution is used. The needle is inserted close to the midline of the wrist anteriorly, distal to the wrist crease and perpendicular to the surface. Superficial veins should be avoided. After traversing the skin and the flexor retinaculum the hydrocortisone is injected. There should be no need to exert pressure; about 0·5 to 0·75 ml is injected. There may be additional discomfort during the subsequent 24 hours. Relief is then usually obtained, but passes off in two or three months.

In mild cases relief may be obtained by applying a splint to support the wrist in mid-position at night.

Ulnar Neuropathy. Transient mild paraesthesiae in the 4th and 5th fingers are common in patients who are ill or disabled, and are attributable to pressure on the ulnar nerve at the elbow. In persistent cases it is helpful to carry out nerve conduction velocity measurements, and localised slowing may be demonstrated at a point of compression, most commonly in the region of the elbow. It may be related to an old fracture of the elbow, osteoarthritis, cyst, recurrent dislocation of the nerve, or local nerve injury. Compression may also present at the wrist, and the deep branch may be compressed in the hand.

More severe cases seldom clear spontaneously, and surgical treatment is by transposition. The standard method is anterior transposition but if it fails, transposition deep to the common flexor origin should be considered. Compression of the deep branch from pressure on the palm usually recovers spontaneously.

Radial Neuropathy. The radial nerve may be compressed in the axilla or as it lies in the spiral groove. It could happen as a complication of fracture or result from the compression associated with heavy sleep or coma. The main disability is wrist drop, but if the lesion is high, power in the triceps may be lost. If continuity of the nerve is retained, recovery usually takes place in three to six months. Relief may be obtained by using a cock-up splint, and contracture must be prevented. If the continuity of the nerve is in doubt, surgical exploration is indicated and suture may be required.

Compression of the posterior interosseus nerve causes finger drop and weakness of wrist extension without sensory loss. It may be compressed between the heads of the supinator muscle or injured close to the elbow. A cyst or lipoma may be associated and will require excision. When the cause is in doubt exploration of the nerve should be considered.

The circumflex nerve may be injured when there is dislocation of the shoulder.

Common Peroneal Nerve Palsy. This causes foot drop, with weakness of eversion of the foot and pain with paraesthesiae and numbness over the dorsum of the foot. The site of neural involvement is usually at the head of the fibula and close to the knee where it is superficial and vulnerable to trauma. The majority recover spontaneously in about three months, and a toe-raising spring provides support during this interval. When a cyst is present it is usually necessary to excise it.

Causalgia. The term was applied by Weir Mitchell to persistent pain following trauma to peripheral nerve. It affects most commonly the sciatic or median nerve and usually the loss of function in the nerve is partial. The pain is of a continuous burning quality and not relieved by simple analgesics. These are trophic changes, and the skin becomes red and shiny. The muscles show atrophy. It has been postulated that nerve impulses may follow an abnormal path via autonomic nerves. In the majority of cases the pain develops within a few hours of the injury.

Sympathectomy offers the best hope of relief, but is not effective in all cases. A temporary sympathetic block is first produced with local anaesthetic. If this gives relief then sympathectomy is performed. When there is no relief from a successful block it is very unlikely that sympathectomy will help.

Femoral Neuropathy. The femoral nerve may be injured by missile or in the course of a surgical operation for femoral hernia. It may be compressed by haematoma, which occurs in patients with haemorrhagic diseases or on anticoagulant therapy. The signs are weakness and wasting of the quadriceps muscles and sartorius with sensory loss over the anterior and medial aspect of the thigh.

Obturator Nerve Palsy. The obturator nerve supplies the adductors of the thigh but a lesion does not cause sensory deficit. The nerve may be involved in disease of the sacro-iliac joint, compression by the fetal head, invasion by malignant tumour or inflammatory disease of the pelvis, injury in fractures of the pelvis, or deformed when a patient is placed in the lithotomy position under anaesthesia.

Tarsal Tunnel Syndrome. This arises when the tibial nerve is compressed by the flexor retinaculum on the medial aspect of the foot. There is numbness or paraesthesiae of the sole with pain and weakness of the intrinsic muscles of the foot. Tenderness may be found below the medial malleolus and digital pressure in that area may reproduce the sensory symptoms. Relief is obtained by surgical division of the retinaculum.

The medial and lateral plantar nerves arise from the tibial nerve and may be involved independently in compression by the flexor retinaculum, or by a ganglion.

In Morton's metatarsalgia a plantar digital nerve is compressed as it crosses the metatarsal head and causes severe pain. A neuroma may form and can be resected.

Surgical Treatment of Mononeuropathy. The term neurotmesis implies section of the nerve so that the ends separate and will not regenerate unless reconstructed. Ideally, primary suture is performed after clean severance, and the axons regenerate and grow distally. The Schwann cells also proliferate and bridge the gap. The rate of growth of the nerve is 1 to 2 mm/day and the end result is less than perfect. If suture is delayed, the distal end of the nerve may shrink and proliferation of Schwann cells may make it necessary to resect more of the severed ends to obtain satisfactory union. Secondary suture is satisfactory within a few months, but if delayed more than six months is more difficult, and the result poor.

Axonotmesis is a result of crushing a nerve. Axons and the myelin sheath are injured, but the stroma remains in continuity. Regeneration takes place at the rate of 1 to 2 mm/day and may be complete. Surgical treatment is not needed.

Neurapraxia is a transient paralysis, due to mild injury, which recovers in a period of hours, days, or weeks. In the more prolonged cases there is injury to the myelin sheath, but the axon remains intact. Nerve conduction can be demonstrated distal to the lesion by clinical testing.

Surgical exploration of peripheral nerves may be indicated when there is laceration, or a missile wound, and function is lost. In traction injuries of the upper limb early exploration of the upper brachial plexus, median, ulnar, and radial nerves may be needed to assess the injury, determine prognosis, and, in the case of the median nerve, to attempt repair. When nerves are injured in association with a fracture of the elbow, the sciatic nerve is involved in a fracture of the hip, or recovery is delayed for more than three months, exploration is desirable. When the nerve is judged to be preserved in continuity, exploration is better avoided at first, but may be needed after a period of months, depending on the length of regeneration required and the time it is likely to take at the rate of 1 mm/day.

18

Motor Neurone Disease, Myasthenia Gravis, and Muscle Disease

These conditions are included together because the lower motor neurone or muscle fibre are primarily involved. In classical motor neurone disease, upper motor neurone involvement is common, but in the chronic spinal muscular atrophies the clinical picture is often difficult to distinguish from muscular dystrophy. The myopathic nature of muscular dystrophy has recently been questioned, and the distinction between primary muscle disorders and spinal muscular atrophy is not as clear cut as is often thought. Many of the conditions dealt with in this chapter are incurable and present a challenge in the management of chronic progressive neurological disease. Myasthenia gravis and polymyositis are treatable although proper management may be difficult. Sophisticated investigations, including detailed electrophysiological studies and muscle biopsy, are frequently required. These should be performed in centres where adequate facilities are available.

CLASSICAL MOTOR NEURONE DISEASE

This is a rapidly progressive disorder, commoner in men, and most frequently seen in the fourth and fifth decades. Three clinical types are recognised: progressive bulbar palsy, amyotrophic lateral sclerosis, and progressive muscular atrophy. The separation of types is frequently blurred. The cause is unknown although the possibility of a chronic virus infection requires serious consideration. Death usually occurs within five years of the onset and earlier when bulbar symptoms predominate.

Diagnosis and Differential Diagnosis. The presence of widespread muscle fasciculation, wasting and weakness, with or without corticospinal tract involvement suggests the diagnosis. If the arms are initially involved, cervical spondylosis, mononeuropathy and peripheral neuropathy require consideration. Sometimes diabetic neuropathy or amyotrophy are mistaken for motor neurone disease. Neuromyopathy resembling motor neurone disease is associated with carcinoma. Presentation with a spastic paraparesis may suggest spinal cord compression or multiple sclerosis. It is usual for the pattern and course of the condition to make the diagnosis obvious.

Investigation. Although the diagnosis is usually made on clinical examination, electromyography demonstrates widespread chronic active denervation. Radiology of the cervical spine and, occasionally, myelography are required. Muscle biopsy is not necessary as a routine. The spinal fluid is normal. Supplementary investigations to exclude diabetes or an underlying carcinoma may be required.

Treatment and Management. Because of the serious nature of the disease it is advisable to admit the patient for a few days for observation and investigation with simple haematology, plain X-rays of the spine, and electromygraphy. If this is done, an opportunity is provided for advising the relatives of the course and prognosis, and they will be satisfied that the condition has been given serious thought.

There is no effective treatment. Various drugs have been tried, including anabolic steroids and pyridostigmine. Pyridostigmine may occasionally produce slight increase in muscle strength and swallowing. Active physiotherapy is frustrating and of no value. It is customary for placebos such as vitamin B12 injections or oral vitamins to be given. These are harmless and have some psychological value.

The patient should be told that he or she has a muscle disorder that is difficult to treat. The bleak prognosis should not be spelled out, but gradual realisation of the situation will develop and then franker discussion is possible. Nevertheless, it is desirable to try to take a positive attitude and changes of harmless medication and genuine interest in hospital follow-up help to maintain hope.

As disability increases a second opinion may be asked for. As in all chronic progressive neurological disease, this should never be denied nor should it result in loss of rapport affecting future care.

Wheelchair existence is ultimately necessary and modifications in the home may be required.

The problem of severe dysphagia presents one of the most difficult aspects of management. Sometimes a tracheostomy with the use of a cuffed endotracheal tube may help severely dysphagic patients who are still ambulant. Cricopharyngeal myotomy may assist dysphagia and is justified under similar circumstances. Eventually, feeding via a nasogastric tube may be required. Procedures such as gastrostomy are of doubtful justification. The object at all times is to relieve suffering. Narcotics can be used as the illness reaches the terminal phase, particularly if there are painful cramps. The usual cause of death is inhalation pneumonia.

Reactive depression and emotional lability are common. In some instances an endogenous depression supervenes and is helped by tricyclic antidepressants.

MYASTHENIA GRAVIS

This is a fluctuating disorder of variable severity. The precise cause is unknown. One explanation is failure of neuromuscular transmission due to defective quanta of acetylcholine at prejunctional sites. The thymus is enlarged, and although the relationship between the thymus and neuromuscular transmission is unknown thymectomy is valuable in the management of the condition. A diagnostic feature of myasthenia gravis is the therapeutic response to anticholinesterase drugs.

Clinical Features. The condition is twice as common in young women but men are more frequently affected in later life. The condition may begin insidiously although sometimes it is of more rapid onset, often related to some specific incident such as trauma or a virus infection. The extrinsic eye muscles are commonly involved, and ocular myasthenia is not uncommon. Bulbar and facial musculature, respiratory muscles and limb muscles are frequently affected. The condition may run a slow fluctuating course but in some instances rapid disability results. A cardinal feature is the daily fluctuation with muscles becoming weaker in the evening. Myasthenia gravis may be associated with thyrotoxicosis. Association with lupus erythematosus, Sjögren's syndrome and rheumatoid arthritis are recorded.

Differential Diagnosis. Myasthenia gravis must be differentiated from primary muscle disorders such as muscular dystrophy and spinal muscular atrophy; the fluctuating symptoms, response to anticholinesterase drugs and fatigability of muscle action potentials in electrodiagnostic studies usually makes this easy. Other neuromuscular disorders may be associated with a neuromuscular transmission defect but this is not prominent. A myasthenic syndrome related to carcinoma known as the Eaton-Lambert syndrome may resemble myasthenia. However, in this disorder muscle power improves with tetanic stimulation, and the reflexes are absent whereas in myasthenia gravis the reflexes are brisk. Post-tetanic facilitation occasionally occurs in true myasthenia gravis.

MANAGEMENT

Medical Treatment. The diagnosis of myasthenia gravis is often confirmed by the intravenous injection of edrophonium chloride (Tensilon) which is a short-acting anticholinesterase drug. An initial dose of 2 mg, followed by the remainder of a 10 mg ampoule if necessary, produces a rapid improvement in muscle power. Care has to be exercised in patients already on treatment and this is discussed below. Negative Tensilon tests do not exclude myasthenia. The neostigmine test may be useful because of the longer action of the drug; 1·5 mg may be injected intramuscularly. Improvement occurs within fifteen minutes and repeated muscle testing may be carried out. Provocative tests using curare are seldom necessary and must not be used without an anaesthetist and resuscitation equipment.

The basis of medical treatment is the use of anticholinesterase drugs to increase the amount of acetylcholine available at the neuromuscular junction. Edrophonium chloride has a very short action and is used only for diagnostic purposes and for assessing whether the patient is undertreated. Neostigminic bromide has a longer action. The 15 mg tablet has a duration of action from two to six hours. The problem with this drug is that the effect may wear off rapidly and require two-hourly administration. There is no fixed dose schedule and the dose requirements may reach 400 to 500 mg a day in divided doses. Pyridostigmine bromide (Mestinon) has a longer and smoother mode of action and is the drug of choice in initial treatment. The dose has to be established by trial and error, and a four-hourly regime is usually satisfactory: 60 mg of pyridostigmine is equivalent to 15 mg of neostigmine. The daily dosage may reach up to 1000 mg or more in some patients. Other anticholinesterase drugs have been used but they are less effective. Ambenomium chloride, bisneostigmine compounds, and alkyphosphates are examples. Ephedrine in a dose of 30 mg t.d.s. is sometimes used but there is little convincing evidence of its value.

Corticosteroids in Myasthenia Gravis. In recent years the value of steroids in myasthenia gravis has become recognised. Courses of ACTH may be used in drug-resistant cases. Originally, the short course of ACTH given on a sliding scale and starting with a 100 i.u. daily was continued for one month. The danger in severe myasthenia is the precipitation of respiratory failure so that the drug should be given to an in-patient with intensive care facilities. There may initially be deterioration, then followed by improvement. Although ACTH has sometimes been regarded as more beneficial than oral steroids, there is no convincing evidence that this is so. Oral corticosteroids are now frequently used and longer regimes adopted. They have been used in the treatment of pure ocular myasthenia gravis with excellent short-term results. The dose regime is arbitrary and is largely a matter of trial. A starting dose of prednisolone 100 mg daily is reasonable and the dose lowered according to the clinical response. Oral corticosteroids are also of value in generalised myasthenia and have been used on a long-term basis, certainly over six months and sometimes longer. There is a vogue for giving prednisolone on alternate days to lessen the side effects. It does appear to be beneficial but some doubt remains about the relative efficiency of this type of regime. Recently short courses of a very high dosage regime have been tried. Methylprednisolone 1 g intravenously daily for five days has proved useful.

Other Immunosuppressive Drugs. Azathioprine, mercaptopurine, and cylophosphamide have all been used. These drugs are relatively untried and their real place in management has still to be decided. Azathioprine in an average dose of 100 mg twice daily is the preferred drug. These drugs should only be used when other methods of medical treatment have failed.

Myasthenic Crisis. A sudden severe increase in myasthenia produces a serious situation and may prove fatal. The important aspect of diagnosis is to distinguish myasthenic crisis from cholinergic crisis. In myasthenic crisis an intravenous injection of 2 mg of edrophonium chloride will improve weakness. An increase in anticholinesterase drugs is then necessary and the patient may require respirator care. Infection, emotional shock, corticosteroids, curare, and streptomycin may precipitate a crisis. However, sudden deterioration takes place as part of the natural disease process.

Cholinergic Crisis. Colic and diarrhoea are common symptoms in patients with anticholinesterase drugs. The symptoms can be controlled by using atropine 0·6 mg three times daily or a similar drug. If cholinergic symptoms such as sweating, miosis, vomiting and pallor occur, an incipient cholinergic crisis can be deduced. If the patient is already taking oral atropine these symptoms may be masked. The nicotinic side effects, namely fasciculation of muscles, will still occur but need not indicate crisis. The pattern of muscle involvement in myasthenia gravis varies, and normal muscles may fasciculate while others are responsive. Cholinergic crisis may be difficult to spot because the patient can pass from a phase of myasthenic weakness to cholinergic weakness without any helpful signs developing. In this situation the edrophonium test can be used but not without intensive care facilities. Crisis may occur in relatively normal muscles such as the respiratory muscles, while limb and eye muscles require larger doses of anticholinergic drugs. Ideally, muscles causing the greatest functional disability should be treated to the maximum but this may be impossible because of cholinergic crisis in other muscles. In assessing muscle strength in response to pyridostigmine or neostigmine it is important to test muscles before and approximately one hour after dosage. It is only by this method that the satisfactory therapeutic dose is reached.

When there is cholinergic crisis the patient often requires assisted respiration and intravenous injections of atropine sulphate, 2 mg at approximately hourly intervals. Signs of atropine toxicity will indicate that enough has been given. It is important not to reintroduce anticholinesterase drugs until the muscles have returned to a myasthenic state. The edrophonium test may be used to assess this. If the patient is on a respirator there is no need to rush the reintroduction of therapy.

THYMECTOMY

The place of thymectomy in the long-term management of myasthenia gravis is established. There is an increasing tendency to operate on patients at an early stage of the disease. One need not wait until drug control is inadequate. Although young women are the most frequent group put forward for operation, men benefit as well. Thymectomy is not used for pure ocular myasthenia because of strict localisation of disability. If the operation is done at an early stage the management is much easier. Medication should be stopped prior to surgery and the vital capacity and the FEV1 on and off medication should be measured. If the vital capacity is below two litres, respirator care is likely to be needed. In most instances nowadays the passage of an endotracheal tube is all that is required. Unless the patient has severe respiratory problems before operation a tracheostomy will not be needed. If the patient is not on a respirator the medication can be reintroduced after the operation at an early stage. There is no urgency if the patient is on assisted respiration. It is usual for the postoperative dose of anticholinesterase drugs to be the same as before the operation.

With regard to the operation itself, the best approach is a sternal split. This allows much better access to the gland than the suprasternal approach, and pericardial fat and other sites for ectopic tissue can be dealt with. It is most important to perform a total removal. Thymectomy is of doubtful value in the presence of a thymoma and even with radiotherapy the prognosis in this group is poor. The beneficial effects of thymectomy are long term and no immediate change may be noticeable. Long-term benefits are a halt in clinical deterioration and gradual improvement often over a period of years.

NEONATAL MYASTHENIA

Children born of myasthenic mothers may have neonatal myasthenia, which is self limiting provided it is recognised and treatment instituted. However, death may ensue because of failure to treat the problem or recognise the possibility. Apart from suction, an injection of 1 mg of edrophonium will improve muscle strength. Pyridostigmine 4 to 20 mg four-hourly may be needed for several weeks. The condition lasts for about three months.

THE EATON–LAMBERT SYNDROME

This is a neuromyopathy that has some features resembling myasthenia gravis, but the electrophysiological findings are different. Certain clinical features are of value. The patient may volunteer that muscle power improves with exercise. The tendon reflexes are usually absent. Tetanic studies show reduced muscle action potentials with single supramaximal stimuli and on tetanic stimulation at 50 Hz there is a small initial decrement in muscle action potential followed by considerable facilitation, as opposed to the decrement usually seen in myasthenia gravis. The disease is usually associated with carcinoma but there are instances when no carcinoma is found over a period of many years.

The treatment is difficult. There is no practical evidence that removal of the cancer or a search for and treatment of metastases helps. Guanidine hydrochloride is the best drug for treating the condition. It is difficult to obtain. A dosage of 20 to 50 mg/kg body weight daily is used in divided doses. Anticholinesterase drugs are not helpful.

MUSCULAR DYSTROPHY AND SPINAL MUSCULAR ATROPHY

These two groups of disorders are considered together as they frequently appear similar from the clinical point of view, and the investigations are the same. Although there is no specific treatment, accurate diagnosis is valuable with regard to prognosis and genetic advice.

Duchenne Muscular Dystrophy. This is taken as the classical type of muscular dystrophy. Other types are mentioned below, but most aspects of management are similar.

Diagnosis and Investigation. The condition develops in the first decade of life. It is inherited as a sex-linked recessive disorder and affects boys. Women are carriers which can frequently be detected by measuring the serum creatine kinase, the simplest and most reliable carrier detection test. The children present with difficulty in walking. They have a waddling gait and frequently show pseudohypertrophy of some muscles, particularly in the calves. Increasing proximal weakness in the legs and arms results in early disability. The diagnosis is made by the age of onset, the clinical findings, a very high serum creatine kinase and electrophysiological and pathological findings. The condition has to be distinguished from spinal muscular atrophy of early onset and rarer muscle disorders that usually have a slower course.

Initial Management. The correct diagnosis is usually obvious clinically although a disorder with slower progression known as the Becker type of muscular dystrophy is similar. The diagnosis requires a full review in the ward, and once this has been completed the nature of the problem has to be explained to the parents.

Carrier Detection. This is an important aspect of management. A female is regarded as a definite carrier if one child and a brother, maternal uncle or male relative on the female side are affected. In the absence of such a family history the presence of two affected children is highly suggestive. The female relatives of the mother with one affected child are possible carriers. The creatine kinase is the most reliable index of confirmation and is raised in 60 per cent of carriers. Electromyography may help in doubtful cases. Muscle biopsy is often not performed but may reveal myopathic changes.

Carrier detection is of little value without appropriate genetic advice.

In the case of a mother with one affected male child, the sex of the fetus can be determined at an early stage and the pregnancy terminated if the fetus is male. In the instance of probable carriers, female relatives with affected sons, the same principle can be applied. The diagnosis in a newborn infant can be made by estimating creatine kinase in cord blood. This provides early information which may be of value in family planning. It is not possible to give overall views about genetic handling of the problem. Each member involved must be seen and the situation discussed individually.

The Ambulant Stage. Duchenne dystrophy presents at about the age of three. At 10 to 12 years of age the boy is usually wheelchair bound. During the period when walking is still possible, every attempt must be made to encourage the child to be active. He should not exhaust himself, but full activity is beneficial and prolongs the ambulant stage. Prolonged rest in bed with intercurrent illness should be avoided. Contractures develop early, in particular in hip flexion and plantar flexion and inversion of the foot. To some extent this can be avoided by regular passive stretching exercises. Nevertheless, in the case of the foot, subcutaneous achilles tenotomy may help the position of the foot. Physiotherapy and leg bracing are needed as well. During the ambulant stage there may be weight gain as a result of lack of activity but this becomes more of a problem in the wheelchair stage. However, it is advisable to keep weight down to reasonable levels at all stages.

It is most important that the child should be subject to normal family life and discipline. This is not easy but the parents' temptation to spoil the child should be resisted. Schooling should be at a normal school if possible. Some children with Duchenne dystrophy have impaired intelligence and may need to be in remedial classes. The geography of the school has some bearing on whether it will remain suitable at the secondary education stage. Absence of staircases and freedom for the use of an electric wheelchair are important.

The Wheelchair Stage. At this stage the child is often glad to give up the struggle of staying on his feet. Even then, the position of the limbs and body is important for comfort. Achilles tenotomy will improve the position of the foot if it has not been done before and will assist in the fitting of shoes. Some degree of scoliosis is inevitable but this can be lessened by attention to proper posture in the chair.

As paralysis increases, chest infections are likely. The heart may be involved. Eventually, death or heart failure ensues around the age of 25, usually from chest infection. Greater attention to physical well being is tending to prolong life.

Specific Treatment. There is no effective medication for muscular dystrophy. Vitamin preparations, amino acids, and anabolic steroids have all been tried. The Muscular Dystrophy Association supports research into the fundamental cause of the disease which, one hopes, will ultimately result in preventative or curative treatment.

DYSTROPHIA MYOTONICA AND OTHER MYOTONIC SYNDROMES

Myotonia occurs in a number of muscle diseases and is the dominant feature in myotonia congenita. Myotonia is the continuing activity of muscle fibres after the voluntary contraction has ceased. The fundamental cause of myotonia is unknown but it is located in the muscle fibre.

DYSTROPHIA MYOTONICA

This condition is inherited as a mendelian dominant, although the degree of clinical expression varies. Apart from the muscle disorder, frontal baldness, cataracts, heart disease, diabetes mellitus, gonadal atrophy, chronic chest disease and dementia may exist.

Weakness and stiffness of the hands is a common presenting symptom. The disease usually starts between the ages of 15 and 20. Bilateral facial weakness, atrophic sternomastoids, dysphagia, wasting and weakness of the forearm muscles, small hand muscles, and anterior tibial muscles produce a characteristic clinical picture. The additional systemic features aid the diagnosis. Myotonia may be elicited in the small hand muscles and the tongue and other limb muscles. In cases with severe weakness, it may be absent.

The rate of progression varies. In patients with a diffuse clinical picture a wheelchair becomes necessary after 20 to 30 years. Inhalation pneumonia, heart failure, or diabetes mellitus may cause earlier morbidity or mortality.

Treatment of Myotonia. If myotonia is functionally disabling there are a number of drugs which reduce it. Their mode of action is unknown. Quinine 300 mg daily and corticosteroids have been used, but at present phenytoin and procainamide are favoured. Phenytoin 100 mg three times daily may be very effective. Procainamide 250 mg four times daily is also helpful. Weakness reduces their effectiveness.

Treatment of other Complications. Visual failure due to cataract may be treated by surgical removal. The chest complications are due to an abnormality of oesophageal motility which causes reflux into the lungs. Chronic bronchiectasis may result and recurrent chest infections require antibiotic therapy. The heart is frequently involved but heart failure is a late complication. It should be treated with digoxin and diuretics.

Genetic Advice. The disease can be diagnosed in the fetus in about 10 per cent of families as there is genetic linkage with the Lutheran blood group and ABH secretor status. Pregnancy can be terminated if examination of amniotic fluid reveals these linkage factors. In practice, this is difficult to put across to parents. Fortunately, fertility is impaired in the condition and the disease may cease to be transmitted. The disease may be detected in the preclinical phase in suspected cases by slit lamp examination and electromyography. This may assist in providing more accurate genetic advice.

Dystrophia Myotonica in Children. The condition can present in infants with bulbar involvement who have difficulty in feeding. It is rare, and there is no effective treatment. In adolescence the condition usually resembles the adult form.

MYOTONIA CONGENITA (THOMSEN'S DISEASE)

This condition is rare. It presents in early childhood but on occasions may not be clinically apparent until the age of ten. Spontaneous improvement comes with age. The condition is usually inherited as a mendelian dominant. A recessive form has been described. In addition to myotonia, widespread muscle hypertrophy is common and the child may resemble an 'Infant Hercules'.

The same drugs are used to treat the myotonia as in dystrophia myotonica. Phenytoin is probably the drug of choice. The clinical response is often excellent. In adult life the treatment can often be withdrawn.

PARAMYOTONIA

In this dominant inherited condition the myotonia is made much worse by cold, although this applies to all types of myotonia to a lesser extent. Cold has to be avoided. The condition may be associated with attacks of periodic paralysis. The usual drugs can be used to treat myotonia, which may occur in the eyelids as well as the limb muscles.

OTHER FORMS OF MUSCULAR DYSTROPHY AND SPINAL MUSCULAR ATROPHY

These conditions have no effective treatment. The points about diagnostic procedures and management are similar to those outlined in the section on Duchenne dystrophy, but a slower course and a different mode of inheritance may apply.

The Becker type of sex linked muscular dystrophy is distinguished from Duchenne dystrophy by its benign course. If there are already affected family members more encouraging information can be given to the parents than in the case of Duchenne dystrophy. If there is only one affected child at the time of diagnosis, the more benign course will be appreciated by prolonged observation. Patients with Becker dystrophy may still be mobile in the 20 to 30 age group.

Limb girdle dystrophy is usually inherited as an autosomal recessive. Dominant and sporadic varieties are described. The commonest age of onset is in the second decade. Deterioration is slower than in Duchenne dystrophy, but the prognosis is worse if the pelvic girdle is involved at the onset. This type of dystrophy may be associated with particular involvement of the quadriceps muscles.

The facioscapulohumeral syndrome may be a primary muscle or a neurogenic disorder. The distinction is made by the usual investigations. The prognosis in either type is better than in Duchenne or limb girdle dystrophy. The condition may progress very slowly and cause little disability until late life.

Various forms of spinal muscular atrophy exist that are difficult to differentiate from muscular dystrophy without detailed investigation. The classical Werdnig-Hoffman type of spinal muscular atrophy in infants is rapidly fatal and there is no treatment. Arrested forms of infantile spinal muscular atrophy are seen that require long-term management. Many of these children are wheelchair bound, but less severe types are met with. The adolescent type of spinal muscular atrophy, the Kugelberg-Welander syndrome is slowly progressive and resembles limb girdle dystrophy.

There are other rare types of muscle disorders such as central core disease, mitochondrial myopathy, myotubular myopathy and nemaline myopathy. They present with a proximal myopathy at an early age and there are no specific facets of management. The diagnosis is based on histological studies, including electron microscopy.

POLYMYOSITIS

Clinical Features and Diagnosis. Polymyositis is an inflammatory disorder of muscle presenting as proximal muscle weakness of acute, subacute or chronic onset. The condition has an immunological basis and may exist on its own with or without skin involvement. It is also associated with lupus erythematosus and other collagen disorders. In this case evidence of systemic disease is apparent. Over the age of 50 nearly half of the cases are associated with an underlying carcinoma.

The diagnosis is easier if there is evidence of other systemic disease. A raised erythrocyte sedimentation rate, protein abnormalities and other disturbances of immunological function help to separate it from spinal muscular atrophy and muscular dystrophy. Muscle biopsy is the most important definitive investigation. It is important to perform the biopsy on a muscle that has not been subject to electromyography. Polymyositis may be confused with myasthenia gravis but the response to edrophonium chloride in myasthenia gravis distinguishes the two conditions.

Treatment. Corticosteroids are the most important aspect of treatment in polymyositis, and prednisolone is the most widely used drug. It is of paramount importance to give high enough doses and for sufficient time. Many failures in therapy are due to inadequate dosage.

The minimum starting dose in an adult is 60 mg daily in a single or divided doses. In some instances 100 mg of prednisolone daily is required. The response to therapy varies with the type of polymyositis. The most favourable response is seen in patients with isolated muscle disease with a rapid onset and early diagnosis. Delay in diagnosis, which may be made several years after the onset, results in slower and incomplete recovery. In the associated collagen disorders the general activity of the disease affecting other organs will influence the outlook. In those patients with associated malignancy the response is usually incomplete and temporary.

There is a vogue for giving prednisolone on alternate days to reduce side effects but this is of dubious value. The patient merely has a lower dose of steroid. Apart from clinical improvement the best index of control is the regular measurement of serum creatine kinase levels. This can be used to assist in the timing of steroid reduction. However, it is common for initial dosage therapy to continue for up to six months. Reduction in dosage must be gradual as relapse is common. Although patients can make an excellent and complete functional recovery they may need to continue indefinitely on 5 to 20 mg of prednisolone daily. In the younger age groups it may be possible to stop steroids after about two years and for remission to continue.

In patients who respond incompletely to steroids or who develop serious side effects, such as severe osteoporosis in middle-aged women, the use of immunosuppressive drugs have been tried. The full value of these drugs is still in doubt. They may be given alone or in combination with steroids. Cyclophosphamide and azathioprine are the simplest agents to use. Azathioprine is used from 50 to 300 mg daily and cyclophosphamide from 100 to 300 mg daily. Side effects need to be looked for by regularly checking the blood picture for haematopoietic suppression. Gastrointestinal upset and hair loss may be experienced in the case of cyclophosphamide.

The place of physiotherapy in the rehabilitation of patients with polymyositis is controversial. Some authorities regard it as valueless, but a course of muscle-strengthening exercises during the phase of recovery is probably of considerable value, particularly in those unaccustomed to physical exertion.

Those patients with polymyositis unresponsive to treatment become problems in the management of chronic progressive muscular disease. The presence of bulbar symptoms are a particular problem and it may be necessary to pass a nasogastric tube. Patients with progressive unresponsive polymyositis often have associated malignant disease and die from the effects of primary or secondary tumours or from lung infection related to the polymyositis.

POLYMYALGIA RHEUMATICA

This is a painful muscle disorder confined to the elderly. The patient complains of aching in the muscles of the upper and lower limbs and may feel generally unwell. Symptoms suggestive of temporal arteritis (page 56) may coexist. Physical examination does not usually reveal muscle weakness but the muscles are tender. The ESR is considerably raised. The treatment is with corticosteroids (*see* page 56). Prednisolone up to 60 mg daily may be used to control the symptoms, and the ESR reflects disease activity. The dose can usually be rapidly reduced to a maintenance level of 10 to 20 mg daily. This may need to be continued for over a year before an attempt at steroid withdrawal can be made.

METABOLIC MUSCLE DISORDERS

A number of myopathies have a known metabolic cause even though the precise effect of the abnormal metabolism may be obscure. Inherited disorders such as familial periodic paralysis are rare. The frequency of some toxic and nutritional myopathies depends on geography and social custom.

Familial Periodic Paralysis. This is a rare group of disorders characterised by attacks of flaccid weakness of the limbs.

Hypokalaemic Periodic Paralysis. In hypokalaemic paralysis the serum potassium falls with the attack although weakness is produced at higher levels than one would expect in normals. The paralysis may last several days. It is best treated by the oral administration of potassium in a dose of 10 to 15 g. Intravenous potassium is not usually necessary. Unfortunately, prophylactic potassium is of no value. The most effective preventative treatment has been acetazolamide in a dose of 250 mg three times daily. Chlorothiazide has been shown to be helpful. It is also important to avoid violent exercises as there may be attacks during rest following violent exertion. As a large carbohydrate intake may precipitate attacks, it is recommended that a low carbohydrate diet with adequate potassium be taken. Attacks lessen with age.

Hyperkalaemic Periodic Paralysis. This condition may be linked with paramyotonia and there may be an associated myopathy. Attacks come on after exercise but are usually shorter than in hypokalaemic paralysis. The periodic attacks are commoner in infancy and childhood. In adults, the myotonia may be more prominent and muscle wasting and weakness may be a permanent feature. The serum potassium rises in attacks.

Prophylactic treatment may be effective. Chlorothiazide in a dose of 500 mg daily is probably the most effective drug. Acetazolamide or dichlorphenamide may also be used.

Malignant Hyperpyrexia. This dramatic disorder is seen in families with subclinical myopathy, which can be detected by measuring serum creatine kinase. The myopathy becomes clinically important when anaesthesia is given. Extreme hyperpyrexia develops and there is muscular rigidity. Unfortunately, prevention is usually only possible when one member of a family has already been affected and the diagnosis can be made by biopsy and measuring the creatine kinase.

Glycogen Storage Disease of Muscle. A number of rare glycogen storage diseases of muscle may be diagnosed in childhood or adult life. They are not treatable, with the possible exception of McArdle's disease due to muscle phosphorylase deficiency. This presents as muscle pain and weakness on mild or moderate exertion, and starts in childhood. Lactate fails to rise during exercise due to an inability to degrade glycogen. The condition is basically benign although a myopathy may develop. Some patients benefit from taking fructose or glucose before exercise but the simplest measure is to avoid severe exercise and live within acceptable limits.

Thyroid Myopathy. A proximal myopathy is associated with thyrotoxicosis. This is distinct from the association of myasthenia gravis with thyroid disease. Weakness and wasting occur. Electromyography may be compatible with a myopathy. Biopsy is frequently unrewarding. The myopathy resolves with treatment of the thyrotoxicosis.

Thyrotoxicosis may be associated with periodic paralysis, particularly in the Far East. It seems that control of thyroid status abolishes the paralytic episodes.

Exophthalmic ophthalmoplegia is the most important form of thyroid myopathy. The patient may appear euthyroid or hypothyroid following treatment. The cause is obscure but the muscle involvement is due to an increase in orbital contents with swelling and infiltration of muscle fibres. The abductors and elevators of the eye are mainly involved. Improvement may be obtained by prescribing large doses of corticosteroids. When exophthalmos is gross, orbital decompression is required (*see* page 182).

Muscle disorders associated with hypothyroidism are less well defined. There is a disorder of muscle contraction as evidenced by myoedema (ridging of muscle on percussion), and the slow contraction and relaxation of muscle when the tendon jerk is elicited. Muscle hypertrophy may ensue with slowness of movement and may be associated with muscle cramps. Treatment of the hypothyroid state resolves these disorders.

Steroid Myopathy. This may be found in association with Cushing's syndrome or as a result of steroid medication. Those resulting from steroid medication are mainly related to steroids containing fluorine, and these drugs should be avoided. The myopathy of Cushing's syndrome resolves when surgical treatment corrects the steroid overproduction. Steroid myopathy from medication is reversible when the drug is withdrawn.

DYSCALCAEMIC MYOPATHY

A proximal muscle disorder has been described in hyperparathyroidism but it does not appear to be related to the level of the serum calcium. There is a similar myopathy in osteomalacia whatever the cause, and the fundamental defect is thought to be related to altered vitamin D metabolism. Dyscalcaemic myopathy must be considered in all patients presenting with proximal muscle weakness and is cured by the administration of vitamin D2 in a dose of up to 15 mg daily. In cases of myopathy associated with parathyroid adenomata the muscle weakness resolves when the tumour has been successfully removed.

19

Infections and Infestations

The management of this group of disorders is now dominated by the selection of appropriate antibiotic therapy. All too often, therapy has been administered before a definite diagnosis has been made or suitable specimens taken for laboratory examination, with the result that it may prove impossible to identify the organism. The term meningo-encephalitis is often used, but for clinical purposes a group of patients with meningitis can be separated from a group with encephalitis although in some instances there is overlap. These two disorders will be discussed separately since their management presents somewhat different problems.

BACTERIAL INFECTIONS

Meningitis. Meningitis must be distinguished from subarachnoid haemorrhage and meningism. In the child, features of meningeal irritation may not be prominent and it is important to carry out a lumbar puncture when there is fever without any apparent cause. In the adult, there will usually be photophobia and headache with neck stiffness, but Kernig's sign is less constant.

Meningitis with Papilloedema. The question of whether or not a lumbar puncture is safe will arise. In the absence of lateralising neurological signs and supported by a normal echo-encephalogram, it is justifiable to perform a lumbar puncture when meningitis is thought to be the diagnosis. Queckenstedt's test is better avoided.

Lumbar Puncture. This procedure may be difficult if the back is rigid. A child may be held in the position of maximum flexion. With an adult it is important to use a firm table or boards across the bed to prevent sagging. We advise intradermal lignocaine 1 per cent and avoid deep infiltration as penetration of the skin is usually the most painful part of the procedure. The needle is inserted at the L5/S1 or L4/5 space in the mid-line with the point directed slightly towards the head. A fine needle is preferred, but if the exudate is thick it may not pass easily through the needle. If no fluid is obtained, suction is applied with a syringe and, occasionally, it may be necessary to use a wider bore of needle. The opening pressure is recorded with the patient in the horizontal position. Fluid contaminated with blood is virtually useless for laboratory examination, and often the fluid clears after a few drops have been removed. If there is difficulty the needle can be inserted one space above or below. Uniformly bloodstained fluid indicates subarachnoid haemorrhage.

Cisternal Puncture. Cisternal puncture is easier than lumbar puncture, but carries the serious risk of damage to the medulla if the needle is inserted too far. A lumbar puncture needle is used with a mark 5 cm from the tip. The neck is shaved to the level of the external occipital protuberance, and the skin cleaned. The patient lies on a firm table, face downwards, and the neck is flexed. The head is supported with sandbags and the procedure explained. The uppermost vertebral spine (C2) is palpated and a small area of skin 1 cm above it in the midline is anaesthetised with 2 per cent lignocaine. The needle is inserted and passed just below the occipital bone. At about 3 cm the ligament offers resistance and the cistern is entered after a further 1 to 2 cm. The needle should not be inserted beyond the 5 cm mark.

Spinal Fluid. If the fluid is uniformly bloodstained or xanthochromic, the diagnosis of subarachnoid haemorrhage is confirmed and little more information can be obtained from it unless it is infected. If the fluid appears clear, it should *not* be assumed than it is normal. We can recall instances where 70/mm^3 cells or protein 7·00 g/litre were associated with clear fluid. A cell count and protein estimation is therefore required urgently in every case when fluid has been obtained. If the specimen is allowed to stand, cells adhere to the tube and the count is inaccurate. When the cell count is raised, staining of smears, culture, and the glucose level will be needed as well.

If the fluid is purulent we advise the administration of 6 mg (10 000 units) of benzyl penicillin intrathecally at the time of the first lumbar puncture. A search is made for organisms in smears and on culture.

A lymphocytic response suggests tuberculosis, viral infection, cryptococcosis, syphilis, leptospirosis, carcinoma, or partially treated bacterial infection. In the early stages of tuberculous meningitis the fluid may contain a high proportion of polymorphs. In the patient with meningitis the cell count in the fluid is likely to be several hundred/mm^3 with a corresponding rise in protein to 2·00 g/litre or more. Spinal fluid glucose levels are lower than blood glucose levels by about 1·7 mmol/litre in the normal. The glucose level may be normal in cases of virus meningitis and parasitic infestation. In tuberculous meningitis it is usually between 1·1 and 1·9 mmol/litre. In pyogenic meningitis glucose is low or absent from the fluid. Meningococci are often intracellular in smears. The importance of attempts to isolate the organism cannot be over-emphasised. There is no more certain guide to the appropriate therapy.

Table 19.1 lists the sulphonamides and antibiotic drugs used in treating infections.

Management of Acute Bacterial Meningitis. In adults and older children the common causes are the meningococcus, pneumococcus, and *Haemophilus influenzae. H. influenzae* is more difficult to identify but diagnosis becomes likely if the other organisms are excluded. *Escherichia coli* is important in neonatal meningitis.

Meningococcal Meningitis. Recovery may come about even without therapy, but the illness is likely to be prolonged and complications may develop. Some strains of meningococci are resistant to sulphonamides, but all are thought to be sensitive to penicillin. It is reasonable to combine the two, giving oral sulphadiazine 100 mg/kg/day four-hourly (3 to 6 g) for an adult and up to 3 g for a child, with benzyl penicillin intramuscularly 150 mg/kg/day (usually 1·75 g to 3 mega units four-hourly). At the outset, intrathecal penicillin 6 mg (10 000 units) may be given as well, but it is seldom necessary to continue with this. The therapy should go on for a week. An occasional complication is circulatory collapse (Waterhouse-Friderichsen syndrome). This may be associated with haemorrhagic skin rash and is due to disseminated intravascular coagulation. Treatment is controversial, but anticoagulant therapy with heparin may be used. Although haemorrhage into the adrenal glands is found at autopsy, the level of circulating cortisol may be normal, and administration of corticosteroids is then ineffective.

Sulphadiazine in a dose of 4 g daily for an adult is an effective prophylactic where it is sensitive to sulphonamide and can be used in controlling an epidemic. It is probably best restricted to outbreaks in closed communities.

Table 19.1. Sulphonamides and Antibiotic Drugs

Drug and dosage unit	*Route*	*Daily dose*	*Intrathecal dose*	*Frequency of administration*	*Duration*
Sulphadiazine 500 mg	oral	100 mg/kg 3–6 g		four-hourly	5–10 days
Co-trimoxazole 480 mg	oral	960 mg		twice daily	5 days
480 mg in 5 ml	i.v.	1920 mg (diluted to 500 ml)		twice daily	5 days
Benzyl penicillin 150 mg/ml	i.m. (i.v.)	150 mg/kg av. 300 mg (500 000 units)	6–12 mg	four-hourly	5–10 days
Procaine penicillin		(As for benzyl penicillin)			
Ampicillin 250 mg	oral	150 mg/kg 2–4 g	3 mg	four-hourly	5 days
Talampicillin		(As for ampicillin—drug is better absorbed than ampicillin)			
Carbenicillin 1–5 g	i.m. (i.v.)	8 g or i.v. 8–30 g by infusion		six-hourly	10 days +
Cloxacillin 250 mg	oral	1 g, child—50 mg/kg		six-hourly	5–10 days
Erythromycin 250 mg	oral	1 g		six-hourly	5–10 days
Tetracycline 250 mg	oral i.m./i.v.	2–3 g 1 g		six-hourly	5–10 days
Chloramphenicol 250 mg	oral	1–3 g	25–50 mg	six-hourly	max. 14 days
1 g ampoule	i.m./i.v.	3–4 g		six-or eight-hourly	

i.m. = intramuscular
i.v. = intravenous

Pneumococcal meningitis. This is a serious condition with a mortality rate that approaches 50 per cent. Penicillin is the drug of choice and should be given both intramuscularly (or intravenously) and intrathecally. The intrathecal dose is 6 mg (10 000 units) daily, for 10 days and the intramuscular 1200 mg (2 mega units) every four hours. If the patient is allergic to penicillin, cephaloridine may be used both intravenously and intrathecally or, alternatively, chloramphenicol.

Haemophilus influenzae Meningitis. The drugs of choice are ampicillin and chloramphenicol. Penicillin is ineffective, but ampicillin has recently emerged as the preferred drug if given intravenously in a dose of 1200 mg (2 mega units) four-hourly at first with intrathecal administration (50 mg) as well. This is probably as effective and less harmful than chloramphenicol which occasionally causes marrow aplasia.

Meningitis in the Neonate. Various organisms cause this condition and Gram-negative bacilli of the *E. coli* type are often found. Symptoms are non-specific and fever may be absent. Mortality is high. While reports of sensitivity are awaited, treatment may be started with ampicillin 150 mg/day intramuscularly and 3 mg intrathecally. Gentamicin 6 mg/kg/day i.m. may be give as well, with 1 mg intrathecally. If this fails, direct instillation of drugs into the ventricles should be considered. Daily doses by this route are gentamicin 1 mg, ampicillin 50 mg, cephaloridine sodium 50 mg, or chloramphenicol 25 to 50 mg used according to sensitivity of the organism.

Other drugs that may be indicated by sensitivity tests include polymixin B sulphate, carbenicillin, and cloxacillin.

Listeria monocytogenes meningitis may be acquired from the mother and is usually sensitive to penicillin.

Other Varieties of Acute Bacterial Meningitis. Meningitis is sometimes a complication of staphylococcal, streptococcal, or *E. coli* septicaemia. In the debilitated patient *Listeria monocytogenes* meningitis may occur. Systemic antibiotics are given according to the sensitivity of the organism. Where treatment is urgent and the exact diagnosis is in doubt, we recommend ampicillin in high dose parenterally. If the patient is sensitive to penicillin, parenteral co-trimoxazole or chloramphenicol may be used. The combination of sulphadiazine, chloramphenicol, and penicillin is no longer necessary.

General Management of the Patient with Meningitis. Intensive care is needed to maintain the physiological state, while specific therapy has time to act. Adequate fluid intake by mouth, gastric tube, or intravenous infusion is essential. When sulphonamide is used, a high urinary output must be maintained to prevent crystalline deposition. A check is kept on the serum electrolyte levels.

Tuberculous Meningitis. The early diagnosis of this condition is difficult and during the first fortnight the spinal fluid may be normal, or may not show the characteristic findings. Polymorphs are commonly present at the beginning and may form a high proportion of the total cells. It is particularly important in this condition to have a thorough search of smears of spinal fluid and the success rate in recovering the organism is related to the experience and application directed to this task. Fortunately, in Europe, tuberculosis is now much less common, but this also means that experience of its diagnosis is more remote. The decision to begin treatment must be dominated by the clinical condition, but in a doubtful case the patient may be better served by delay in administering antibiotics while several specimens of spinal fluid are examined, than by commitment to a complicated course of prolonged therapy. Table 19.2 gives a list of drugs and regimes used in the treatment of tuberculosis.

The most effective drugs in the chemotherapy of tuberculosis are isoniazid, streptomycin, ethambutol, rifampicin, pyrazinamide, ethionamide, and para-aminosalicylic acid. The last-named should probably now be discarded as it is generally found unpalatable by patients and is less effective than the others. It would be generally agreed that these drugs should not be used singly, and it is common practice to administer three drugs initially until the sensitivity of the organism is known from culture, which takes several weeks. The initial regime might then be streptomycin 1 g daily intramuscularly with isoniazid 300 to 600 mg daily by mouth with pyridoxine 10 mg (page 249) and ethambutol 15 mg/kg per day or, alternatively, rifampicin 450 to 600 mg/day before breakfast. Chemotherapy will need to be continued for a minimum of one year. The development of resistance to drugs is much reduced by using them in combination, and some people prefer to make a change in the regime at intervals of, say three months, combining the different pairs, provided the organism is known to be sensitive (*see* Table 19.2). The possibility of tuberculosis elsewhere must be borne in mind, and may require modification of the regime.

In the child, the regime outlined above in modified dosage may prove sufficient to control this disease. In adults, the condition tends to be more difficult to manage, and some of the most virulent cases of all are seen in immigrants. If the patient is in a serious condition, or if after a week there is little evidence of response to a regime of treatment, the possibility of

Table 19.2. Tuberculosis—Drugs and Regimes

Drug and dosage unit	*Activity*	*Toxicity*	*CSF penetration*	*Dose (adult)*
Isoniazid 50 mg; 100 mg	high	low	good	oral 300–600 mg/day with pyridoxine 10 mg
Streptomycin 1 g	high	depends on renal function	poor except where meninges inflamed	i.m. 1 g daily Intrathecal 100 mg daily
Ethambutol 100 mg *400 mg*	high	low if dose below 15 mg/kg/day and full renal function	when meninges inflamed	oral 15 mg/kg/day
Rifampicin 150 mg 300 mg	high	low; hepatic	high	oral 300–600 mg/day, one dose before breakfast
Pyrazinamide 500 mg	moderate	high; hepatic, secondary gout	good	oral 25 mg/kg/day
Ethionamide 125 mg	moderate	high; hepatic, nausea	good	oral 0·75–1 g daily

Regimes:

1. Isoniazid + streptomycin + prednisolone   low toxicity   not bactericidal
   or
   ethambutol
2. Isoniazid + streptomycin + rifampicin
   or
   Ethionamide   ethambutol
3. Isoniazid + rifampicin + pyrazinamide for two months
   then
   Isoniazid + rifampicin

other measures must be considered.

Intrathecal streptomycin is not favoured by paediatricians, and controlled trials leave some doubt whether anything is gained by its use. Some clinicians have been impressed with the response of apparently resistant cases when this therapy is introduced, and we would certainly advise it in such a situation. The dose of intrathecal streptomycin is 100 mg daily for an adult (50 mg for a child) and it should be continued for at least three weeks. Provided the clinical course of the patient is satisfactory, the persistence of a raised cell count in the spinal fluid of the order of 20 to 30 lymphocytes is not necessarily an indication to use intrathecal treatment, but such a case will need to be followed up carefully and the spinal fluid re-examined at intervals of a month or six weeks. Intrathecal streptomycin may cause a pleocytosis.

The use of corticosteroid therapy either systemically or intrathecally is also controversial. It may control inflammatory exudate and, provided adequate chemotherapy is given at the same time, this should result in a general improvement. There is evidence that the use of corticosteroids may prevent the development of a spinal block or even help when one has developed. Oral prednisolone 60 mg daily for an adult may be given in the acute stage of the disease or at any time when the spinal fluid protein is high or shows signs of rising. It may then be appropriate to use intrathecal hydrocortisone 50 mg daily as well.

The use of intrathecal tuberculin is more controversial. There is some evidence that in severe and resistant cases, the treatment may be beneficial, and it should certainly be considered when other regimes are failing to control infection. Most of the work on this has been done at Oxford (Smith *et al.*, 1956), and experience of it elsewhere is very limited. The object is to cause a tuberculin reaction in the spinal fluid by using progressively higher doses.

The initial response to a regime of treatment is often satisfactory provided that the full dosage is given. The development of new neurological signs indicate that treatment is inadequate. It may be possible to control the situation by adjustment of dosage but if hydrocephalus has developed a shunt may be needed. If the patient is discharged, a very careful supervision must be maintained to ensure that drugs are being taken and that progress is satisfactory. Spinal fluid examination must be repeated until it is normal, which may take several months.

It is currently fashionable to rely on modern drug regimes without intrathecal therapy and other supplementary measures. Some patients who fail to improve find their way to Neurological Units.

Prognosis in Tuberculous Meningitis. Previously fatal, tuberculous meningitis remains a serious disease, but the prognosis for survival has improved with modern therapy. Even those in coma may respond. Mortality should be less than 20 per cent, but is higher in those under three years of age. Development of hydrocephalus and severe neurological deficit are unfavourable.

Morbidity is significant. Mental deficiency, psychiatric disorder, visual loss, deafness, hydrocephalus, and convulsions may complicate the clinical state, but above 70 per cent are able to lead a normal life.

Tuberculoma and Pott's Paraplegia. A tuberculoma may arise in the brain or spinal cord. It is rarely seen in the United Kingdom, but is most likely to be located in the posterior fossa in a patient under 40. Chemotherapy should be instituted, and although some cases respond most require surgical excision as well. Results are good, about 70 per cent make a complete recovery.

In Pott's disease the initial measure is chemotherapy and this is continued for a year or longer. Surgery is required when paraplegia develops suddenly or neurological deficit increases in spite of chemotherapy.

Lateral or anterior decompression and excision may be carried out or laminectomy if there is spinal compression.

Syphilitic Meningitis. This is now a rare condition, but worth considering in those with a lymphocytic meningitis. The serological tests will confirm the diagnosis and the treatment of choice is benzyl penicillin.

Carcinomatous Meningitis. Patients with metastatic tumour involving the meninges or with microglioma may show lymphocytosis in the spinal fluid with raised protein and low glucose. The fluid therefore resembles that found in tuberculous meningitis. Headache and other signs of meningitis may be absent. The tumour may be identified as cells in spinal fluid. Treatment is unsatisfactory.

Recurrent Meningitis. This is uncommon, and its occurrence must raise the possibility of some predisposing factor. Among the causes that have been reported are meningomyelocele, congenital dermal sinus, skull defects, and, rarely, an ulcer of the sacrum may become infected and cause meningeal inflammation. There is also the problem of the patient with cerebrospinal otorrhoea or rhinorrhoea which may follow trauma to the head or a surgical procedure.

Rhinorrhoea in particular is liable to lead to meningeal infection. If it does not cease spontaneously within a few weeks, the defect must be defined and closed. Prophylactic antibiotic therapy should be used during this period.

Chronic Meningitis. This is also uncommon, but occasionally presents difficulties in both diagnosis and treatment. Among the recognised causes may be noted mycobacteria, enteric organisms, brucellosis, Q fever, *Cryptococcus neoformans* (torulosis), and *Coccidia immunitis*. Confirmation of the diagnosis will usually depend on culture of the spinal fluid.

Meningitis Associated with Reticulosis and Leukaemia. The use of potent drugs in the treatment of leukaemia and reticulosis has increased the length of survival and also the frequency of meningeal involvement which has now become relatively common. Many of these patients are now treated with a combination of corticosteroids and immunosuppressive drugs, and the latter often prove to be toxic to the marrow and other tissues.

Meningeal leukaemia is common in children with acute lymphoblastic leukaemia. It may develop while control of the disease is otherwise adequate, but it is often the prelude to a general deterioration. Early diagnosis of the meningeal involvement is important and a case is made for prophylactic radiation of the cranium combined with intrathecal methotrexate 6 mg/m^2 every four weeks for ten months. This treatment increases the duration of the remission and life may be prolonged for more than five years. In myelogenous leukaemia, involvement of the central nervous system is less common, and treatment, although similar to the lymphoblastic type, is less firmly established.

BRAIN ABSCESS

Whenever there are features of encephalitis the possibility of bacterial infection with suppuration must be considered. Usually, there is a predisposing factor such as septicaemia, otitis, lung abscess, bronchiectasis, sinusitis, or a recent head injury. There is usually a delay of several days before the abscess develops. It may present with epilepsy, alteration in behaviour or psychosis, drowsiness, confusion, or coma. Fever and toxaemia may be combined with focal neurological signs and papilloedema. Examination with the auriscope is important. Signs of meningeal irritation are usually absent. The spinal fluid shows a slight increase in lymphocytes or polymorphs up to about $30/mm^3$, slight rise in protein, and normal glucose level. The electroencephalogram may show diffuse slow wave activity at about 1 a second with focal changes. The isotope brain scan or computerised axial tomogram will demonstrate the lesion.

Treatment consists, in the first instance, of prevention by dealing with the predisposing factors. The presence of focal epilepsy or focal neurological signs will always suggest abscess and usually indicate further investigation. Cerebral abscess does not respond to antibiotic therapy alone, and must be regarded as a surgical emergency. When a localised lesion has been demonstrated, the surgeon will usually make a burr hole and explore with a needle with a view to aspiration. The aspirate should be cultured aerobically and anaerobically. If fluid is aspirated, then a small quantity of Myodil is injected, which will make it possible to observe subsequent progress with plain radiographs. Repeated drainage may be needed and a course of antibiotic therapy is given at the same time. When a satisfactory response is obtained it is important to deal with the predisposing cause since the development of one brain abscess predisposes to a further episode later. This particularly applies to middle ear and sinus infection. On the second occasion, the signs of abscess developing may be much less obvious. Brain abscess carries a mortality of 50 per cent, even in the best managed cases. It may be improved by earlier diagnosis. The question of radical excision of the abscess is controversial. There can be little place for this in the acute stage, but some surgeons advise it after the infection has been controlled, while others consider it unnecessary.

Subdural, Extradural and Parafalcine Abscess. These are most likely to develop in the presence of sinus or ear infections and are surgical emergencies. Pain, tenderness, epilepsy, toxaemia, features of raised intracranial pressure, and focal signs (commonly hemiplegia) may all be present. Burr holes and drainage are required. They most often occur in children.

Spinal Epidural Abscess. In this uncommon condition severe pain in the back and localised tenderness are associated with signs of spinal compression and toxaemia. The evolution is rapid and surgical drainage is urgently required.

Cortical Thrombophlebitis. This also arises as a complication of trauma or infection in the ear or paranasal sinuses. Headache, toxaemia, raised intracranial pressure and epilepsy are common findings. Treatment consists of intensive antibiotic therapy combined with relief of intracranial pressure by surgical methods.

SYSTEMIC BACTERIAL INFECTIONS THAT INVOLVE THE NERVOUS SYSTEM

Tetanus. This infection is due to contamination of wounds and is more common in rural areas. The danger comes from absorption of toxin, which may cause death or severe effects on the neuromuscular junctions and on the autonomic nervous system.

Prophylactic tetanus toxoid is now given routinely to children in Great Britain and a booster dose can be administered if there is exposure to infection. The other important measures are excision of the wound, use of penicillin, and the general management. Adequate attention to the wound must always be given. If not previously immunised a dose of human gamma globulin is usually considered adequate for an adult. Penicillin is advised intramuscularly. The case that evolves rapidly is likely to have a poor prognosis, while the one that develops slowly may recover even though a diagnosis is not made. Provided the patient can be tided over the acute stage, ultimate recovery is likely. Adequate management calls for all the resources of intensive care. Tracheostomy and artificial respiration are discussed in Chapter 1. Tubocurarine may be used to control muscle spasm. Chlorpromazine is useful. At the same time, it is vital to ensure that the fluid intake is adequate, feeding is maintained, and the skin is protected from ulceration by turning the patient frequently. It may be necessary to go on with this intensive care over a period of weeks. Few conditions call for more skill and perseverance in management. When tachycardia is persistent, a beta blocking agent such as propranolol may be helpful. Hypotension may be due to autonomic effects. It may be of abrupt onset and sudden termination, and triggered off by aspiration of secretions or other environmental stimuli. The situation can be controlled by tilting the patient, or by adding dead space to the patient's airway, and so producing a rise in arterial pCO_2.

Leptospirosis. This may cause lymphocytic meningitis, encephalitis, or myelitis. Farmers, dairy staff, abattoir workers and meat processors are at risk. The initial illness is often meningitis and the kidney may be involved. The organism may be seen by dark ground microscopy of blood, urine, or spinal fluid, and then cultured. Serological tests may help. All strains are responsive to penicillin if given early, and a week's course of benzyl penicillin intramuscularly 1200 mg daily is adequate.

Diphtheria. Diphtheria is now rare in Europe because active immunisation is widely used. In those not previously immunised, antitoxin in a dosage of 20 to 100 000 units is given as early as possible. The organism is sensitive to penicillin, but as an alternative, erythromycin can be used. Corticosteroid therapy may be of some value if the patient is shocked. The neurological effects can be considered in three stages. In the acute stage of faucial diphtheria the local effect of toxin may cause a palatal palsy. After about 10 days accommodation of the eye may be affected. The third stage is reached after several weeks when the patient may develop a Guillain-Barré type of neuropathy. The problem in this disease is the control of toxaemia in the acute stage. Although the organism is readily controlled with antibiotics the production of even a small amount of toxin may lead to death from heart failure.

Enteric Fever. Meningitis is a rare complication of typhoid fever and occurs in about 0·1 per cent of the cases. The serious effects of this illness have been offset by antibiotic therapy and the use of prophylactic TAB inoculation. Chloramphenicol is effective, and has the added advantage that it penetrates the blood-brain barrier. A fortnight's course is usually advised, giving 3 g daily to an adult in the febrile state, later reducing to 2 g daily to complete the course over a period of 14 days. The drug may be given orally or intravenously if the patient cannot tolerate oral therapy. There is evidence that some strains of bacilli are resistant to chloramphenicol. Ampicillin is less effective, but it now seems that co-trimoxazole is of comparable value. It should be given over the course of a fortnight.

Botulism. This is now rare. The toxin acts at the neuromuscular junction. The spores are heat-resistant and the infection is usually acquired by eating contaminated meat. Because of its rarity the value of active immunisation is limited, but it is worth considering for laboratory workers. In the acute illness the value of antitoxin is doubtful. If the sub group is known, a monovalent antitoxin may be used. Otherwise, the trivalent preparation covering A B and E can be given in a dose of 100 000 units intravenously. Antibiotics have no specific effect. The general management of the patient is important and will usually require tube feeding, tracheostomy and, sometimes, artificial respiration. Guanidine is reported to be of some value.

Syphilis. Neurosyphilis is now rare in Europe and the milder forms may be overlooked. When there is no history of infection and the clinical features do not suggest the disease the full range of serological tests should be applied to blood and spinal fluid. The cell count in spinal fluid is the most useful index of disease activity. The pathology may be predominantly meningovascular or parenchymatous. The drugs of choice are (*a*) benzyl penicillin, (*b*) tetracycline, and (*c*) erythromycin.

There is some risk from a Jarisch-Herxheimer reaction and this has been ascribed to the toxin derived from sudden destruction of spirochaetes. Attempts to avoid this by using small doses of penicillin initially have not proved successful. The course advised is 600 mg (600 000 units) daily for 10 days of procaine penicillin intramuscularly. Corticosteroids may be used to control a sensitivity reaction. If the patient is known to be sensitive to penicillin, one of the other drugs is used. There is no need for intrathecal therapy.

Leprosy (Hansen's Disease). The acid-fast bacillus that causes this disease commonly invades peripheral nerve and Schwann cells and so causes weakness, wasting, pain, sensory loss, trophic change and thickening of the nerves. Patients with poor resistance may develop the lepromatous type of disease, and the tuberculoid type is seen when resistance is high but incomplete. These types therefore represent the ends of a spectrum of disease. The bacillus may be identified in tissue smears. BCG vaccination is partially effective in prevention.

Treatment is usually with dapsone by mouth. The initial dose for an adult is 25 mg weekly for 4 weeks; then 50 mg weekly for 4 weeks; after which it is increased from 100 to 300 mg. Treatment is continued for two to four years. In resistant cases clofazimine 100 mg three times a week or rifampicin may be used.

When there are skin reactions or erythema nodosum leprosum develops, corticosteroid therapy is helpful. Thalidomide up to 25 mg daily was reported to be very effective in erythema nodosum leprosum. Preliminary results with transfer factor are favourable.

Pain may respond to these measures together with simple analgesics. In severe cases surgical decompression of the nerve sheath is sometimes advised. Physiotherapy and general nursing measures relieve skin ulceration. When infection is controlled, orthopaedic procedures such as tendon transplant may restore function. The central nervous system is spared.

VIRAL INFECTIONS OF THE NERVOUS SYSTEM

Many virus infections are self-limiting in their effects, and it is often difficult to identify the organism. Virus particles contain nucleic acid and multiply within cells. The successful culture of the virus requires cellular material, and this limits its application in the nervous system. The effect of virus on the nervous system is closely related to immunity responses, and in some instances an allergic type of reaction may be the dominant part of the illness. Few drugs are active against viruses, and their use is limited by toxic effects on the cell. Vaccination is an effective method of inducing active immunity, and in the case of rabies it can be used after the infection has been acquired. It has long been appreciated that viruses may cause acute illness such as poliomyelitis, but the concept of a chronic virus disease is more recent.

Diagnosis. Culture may be obtained from spinal fluid, or brain, but when the infection is generalised other tissues may be available. Serum antibody is useful, but since a rise in titre must be shown it takes several weeks to obtain the result. The immuno-fluorescent antibody technique may facilitate identification in tissue. Histological examination may show inclusion bodies, and the virus may be seen by electron microscopy.

Antiviral Drugs. Idoxuridine (5-iodo-2′-deoxyuridine) interferes with DNA synthesis and is only effective against DNA virus such as herpes simplex. As a topical application to the cornea, it is valuable in the treatment of herpes simplex keratitis. In systemic infection it must be given intravenously, and is much less effective. This is partly because of the toxic effect on marrow and liver which limits dosage. It commonly causes stomatitis and alopecia. It now seems doubtful whether the use of the drug in encephalitis is justified by the results obtained.

Amantadine can be administered by mouth and is well absorbed. It is useful in the prevention of A2 influenza, but ineffective against type B influenza and measles. The dose is 200 mg daily. It seldom causes toxic effects, but should be avoided in pregnancy and in patients with epilepsy and arteriosclerosis.

Methisazone is a thiosemicarbazone and interferes with RNA. It can be given by mouth. It is effective against the pox group of viruses and most useful in variola minor. Variola major is much less certain in its response. The main toxic effect is vomiting. A course usually consists of 3 g daily for 4 days followed by 6 g daily for a further 4 days.

Cytarabine arabinoside inhibits nucleoside reductase and DNA polymerase. Its place in the management of herpes zoster remains uncertain. In herpes simplex infection it can be given orally and intrathecally. The usual course is 7 days treatment with 70 mg a day by mouth and 15 mg intrathecally. It may cause gastrointestinal upset and suppress immunity. It is also toxic to liver and marrow. Trials in herpes simplex encephalitis are continuing.

Management of Viral Encephalitis. Many of the milder types of virus encephalitis probably go unrecognised, and they are common during influenzal epidemics. The occurrence of encephalitis in the course of measles, rubella, mumps, or other specific infection will be recognised as a complication and only rarely is it a presenting feature of the disease.

Encephalitis of viral origin must be distinguished from bacterial infection such as tuberculosis, brain abscess, hemiplegic migraine, toxic effects due to drugs and poisons (such as lead in children), and metabolic disorders such as liver failure and porphyria. Differentiation is based on the clinical history, physical examination, examination of spinal fluid, echoencephalogram, EEG, isotope brain scan, computerised axial scan, and sometimes brain biopsy. Virus may be cultured from cellular material. Usually, the organism cannot be identified in the first few days and when serological tests are used the diagnosis is retrospective.

Viral encephalitis is commonly due to arbor or echo virus, but the most severe type is associated with herpes simplex. This variety will be described to illustrate the points in management.

Herpes Simplex Encephalitis (necrotising encephalitis). This condition is associated with high mortality. It may evolve rapidly. Headache, vomiting, and drowsiness are common. The patient is febrile and toxic. Focal or generalised epileptic attacks may occur. Progression to coma is common and there may be signs of neurological deficit or raised intracranial pressure. If the second week is survived, there may be recovery, but residual neurological damage is common.

Spinal fluid examination usually shows a slight increase in cells and protein. The EEG usually demonstrates slow (delta) rhythms of the order of 1 a second and may reveal focal change. The temporal lobes are commonly involved.

Precise diagnosis is difficult. The possibility of brain abscess must always be considered and if focal signs develop, further radiological examination may be needed.

The question of *brain biopsy* arises because it is the only method of confirming the diagnosis. It is certainly justified if the diagnosis is in real doubt. The non-dominant temporal lobe is the preferred site for biopsy. Precautions are necessary to avoid contamination of the specimen during or after removal. Immunofluorescent techniques provide a rapid diagnosis.

Management. The principles can be considered under five headings—

1. *Control of Epilepsy.* This is urgent and it is better to avoid using sedatives. Phenytoin can be given by mouth, gastric tube, or intravenous-

ly. It is advisable to check the serum level and this is also helpful when the route of administration is changed. In more urgent cases intravenous diazepam 20 mg followed by a slow intravenous infusion of 100 mg every 12 hours is satisfactory. This drug suppresses the EEG discharge.

2. *Intensive Care is Essential.* Care of the mouth, skin, fluid balance, and nutrition are basic, and if the patient is in coma, tube feeding and catheterisation will be required. Assisted respiration is occasionally indicated.

3. *Anti-viral Agents.* None is of proved value. Intravenous idoxuridine has been widely used, but is of doubtful value and produces severe toxic effects. Cytarabine is less toxic and can be given orally 70 mg/day with 15 mg intrathecally. The course is continued for a week. The results are uncertain, and trials continue.

4. *Corticosteroid Therapy.* This is the most effective means of controlling brain oedema, which is a serious problem. It can be given intravenously or by mouth as dexamethasone 4 to 20 mg daily. It must be continued through the acute stage of the illness.

Reservations have been expressed about the wisdom of using corticosteroid therapy in the presence of uncontrolled infection. In general, it would seem that the risks are outweighed by the importance of controlling brain oedema.

5. *Antibiotic Therapy.* While ineffective against the virus, these drugs have an important place in the control of secondary bacterial infection of the chest or bladder, particularly in the comatose patient. It is reasonable to administer a broad spectrum antibiotic such as ampicillin 1 to 2 g daily. If culture of secretions reveals an organism that is sensitive, then the appropriate antibiotic is given.

In herpes simplex encephalitis the mortality is about 80 per cent.

Rabies. The mortality in this disease is very high, and only rare instances of survival are reported. Quarantine regulations for import of animals have kept it under control, but in Europe it is spread by foxes, dogs, vampire bats and other mammals. The incubation period is usually about six weeks but can be up to a year. Three measures are important in dealing with a patient exposed to rabies from a bite; thorough excision of the wound, local application of antitoxin, and vaccination. Active immunisation with a duck embryo preparation requires a course of sixteen injections given into the anterior abdominal wall. It is not always effective.

Encouraging results have been reported with human diploid cell vaccine (HDCV). There is a high antibody response and few reactions. It is given intradermally at intervals of a few days. The regime is not yet established but three injections may be sufficient. It may prove to be of prophylactic value.

Herpes Zoster. This disorder is most familiar as a vesicular eruption following a nerve root distribution and associated with infection of the root ganglion. It may represent reactivation of varicella. There is pain, and secondary infection may be added. When the cranial nerves are affected the first division of the trigeminal is commonly involved. The disease is more widespread than the signs would suggest. There may be motor involvement which is sometimes permanent. A Guillain-Barré syndrome is sometimes associated with herpes zoster.

A slight rise in cells and protein in the spinal fluid is common, but clinical features of meningo-encephalitis are rare. Occasionally there is a myelopathy.

Calamine lotion and antihistamines are useful in managing the skin eruption. If idoxuridine is applied locally as a 40 per cent solution in dimethyl sulphox, using lint soaked in the solution and held in position by bandages for 4 days (changed every 4 hours), pain is relieved, but the treatment is expensive. It should not be used in pregnancy, and there is a smell of garlic.

Systemic corticosteroid therapy has been advised. If used early, it may give relief of pain and shorten the illness. There is some risk of extension of the skin lesion. Local application of corticosteroid cream is less effective and contra-indicated because of spread of vesicles and subsequent scarring.

Secondary infection may be due to *Staphylococcus aureus* and can be controlled with local application of fucidic acid or gentamicin. In ophthalmic herpes, local idoxuridine is useful (plastic spectacle frames dissolve in dimethyl sulphox). Oedema around the eye usually clears in a few days. Careful observation of the eye is essential and any sign of inflammation should be an indication for dilatation of the pupil using 1 per cent atropine eye drops.

There is no established systemic chemotherapy. Amantadine has been used, but is ineffective.

Poliomyelitis. This disease is now rare. An important factor in reducing the incidence is the successful use of vaccine. Live attenuated vaccine is usually given in 3 doses at six months, nine months, and one year of age. The picorna (RNA) virus occurs in three strains and there is little cross-immunity.

The initial (minor) illness is non-specific and settles in a few days. There may then be a meningitic phase. As the major illness develops, pain is severe and there may be paralysis, which does not progress after the fever settles. If there is bulbar or diaphragmatic involvement, assisted respiration may be needed. Acute retention of urine may require relief by catheterisation. Intensive care is important. There is no effective chemotherapy. The place of corticosteroid therapy has not been defined.

Rehabilitation may have to be prolonged. Natural recovery is sometimes remarkable. When the situation has stabilised the possibility of tendon transplant and other orthopaedic procedures must be considered. Urinary calculi may form in the immobile.

Infectious Mononucleosis (Epstein-Barr virus). Involvement of the nervous system is uncommon. A lymphocytic meningitis, encephalitis, acute myelopathy, or radiculopathy may occur. Facial diplegia and respiratory failure have been reported. There is no specific therapy.

Cytomegalic Virus Infection. This shows a clinical resemblance to infectious mononucleosis, and also to toxoplasmosis (page 236). It is probably a DNA virus which induces a giant cell reaction in the host. The congenital type, which is acquired in utero, and the infection in patients who are immunologically suppressed carries a poor prognosis.

NEUROLOGICAL DISORDERS ASSOCIATED WITH SPECIFIC FEVERS

These are uncommon and develop in less than 5 per cent of patients with measles, mumps, varicella. Similar manifestations are seen after vaccination against rabies and smallpox.

Two types are usually distinguished. One, which usually develops early in the course of the exanthem, is due to direct invasion of the nervous system by the organism. The second type is regarded as an allergic response and characteristically develops 10 to 14 days from the onset. From the clinical point of view there is some overlap of the two groups, although the pathological mechanisms are distinct.

Encephalopathy is the commonest manifestation, but myelopathy and radiculopathy also occur. The clinical presentation may take any of these forms; often one predominates but components of the others are also present. The majority recover, but recovery may be slow and take many months. Death sometimes ensues in those with encephalitis, particularly the type associated with measles.

The management in general is that of coma or any encephalopathy. Corticosteroid therapy in moderate dosage such as 60 mg of prednisolone daily for an adult is advised in the allergic type. If this treatment is used early in the illness the rash may recur and there is some risk of spread of the virus, although this is probably not serious.

Subacute Sclerosing Panencephalitis. This uncommon disorder is usually found in children and adolescents. It begins with ill-defined psychiatric symptoms and changes in behaviour. Over a period of months, there is deterioration and mental functions show impairment. There may be signs of disease of nerve pathways. It has recently been shown that the measles virus is responsible. Occasionally there is spontaneous arrest, but usually the condition progresses over two or three years to cause death. Recently, treatment with amantadine, transfer factor, and splenectomy has been tried, but none can yet be said to be established.

OTHER INFECTIONS OF THE NERVOUS SYSTEM

Mycoses. Mycoses of the nervous system may be found in people with a past history of local fungal infection, or as part of a systemic disturbance. It is particularly likely to arise in the debilitated patient with some other disease. Meningitis or encephalitis may be caused.

The diagnosis may be made by examination of the spinal fluid, which is sometimes xanthochromic. The cell count seldom exceeds 1000 mm^3 and special stains are needed to identify the organism. Both anaerobic and aerobic cultures should be set up. Skin tests and serological tests may help. Histological examination may also be useful as, for example, when material is obtained by aspiration of the brain when seeking an abscess.

The identification of the fungus is a specalised matter. Those that invade the nervous system include actinomycosis which may spread from the jaw to the meninges, aspergillosis which may spread by the blood to the brain, and cryptococcus (torulosis) which particularly attacks the debilitated.

The most useful drug is amphotericin B. This therapy is indicated in blastomycosis, histoplasmosis, *Cryptococcus neoformans*, candida and sporotrichosis. It is not effective in aspergillus infection. It is not well absorbed from the gut, but can be given parenterally; 50 mg dissolved in water and thoroughly shaken is then diluted with 5 per cent glucose so that the concentration is less than 10 mg per cent. The daily dose of 1 mg/kg to a maximum of 50 mg given in six hours is continued for about six weeks. Renal function must be checked and hypokalaemia corrected. Muscle weakness or cardiac arrhythmia may develop. This intravenous therapy may be supplemented by intrathecal doses of 0·5 mg in at least 5 ml two or three times a week.

In *Cryptococcus neoformans* an alternative drug is flucytosine in a dosage of 150 mg/kg/day by mouth. It is less toxic than amphotericin, but may cause a fall in the white cell or platelet counts, nausea, hepatic dysfunction, and vertigo.

Malaria. Cerebral malaria is a disease of young children in endemic areas but affects visitors of any age who may develop it several weeks after leaving the endemic zone. It commonly presents with epilepsy or coma and is a medical emergency. *Plasmodium falciparum* may be seen in thick stained blood films. The spinal fluid is normal. Treatment consists of intensive care, intravenous fluids, and antimalarial drugs.

Intravenous quinine hydrochloride 600 mg in 25 ml of physiological saline should be given six hourly at first and combined with a course of chloroquine sulphate 600 mg orally and then 300 mg every twelve hours for 3 days. As an alternative to quinine chloroquine sulphate 200 to 300 mg can be given intravenously.

Prophylaxis is with proguanil (100 to 200 mg daily), chlorproguanil 20 mg weekly, or pyrimethamine 25 to 50 mg weekly.

Toxoplasmosis. Infection with *Toxoplasma gondii* is common but the clinical disease is rare. An infection in the mother may spread via the placenta to the fetus. This may lead to stillbirth or survival with involvement of eye or brain.

In the adult, acquired infection rarely leads to encephalitis except in those with disorders of immunity. The diagnosis is based on serological tests. Treatment is usually with spiramycin 2 to 3 g daily for six weeks or pyrimethamine 25 mg daily combined with a sulphonamide. Folate deficiency may develop and corticosteroids are useful in controlling sensitivity reactions that may arise when active disease is present.

Amoebiasis. Entamoeba is responsible for this condition which begins in the intestine. Abscesses may form in the liver and lung and, more rarely, in the brain. Systemic treatment may be with emetine and chloroquine, but metronidazole 400 to 800 mg t.d.s. for 10 days is the treatment of choice.

Cysticercosis. The cystic phase of *Taenia solium* may occur in the brain or spinal cord. This is common in India and South America. Epilepsy may be the presenting feature several years after infection. Occasionally, raised intracranial pressure, mental symptoms, or features of spinal compression develop. It may cause pseudohypertrophy of muscle, and radiographs of muscle may show cysticerci.

Treatment is unsatisfactory. Epilepsy may respond to anticonvulsants. Obstructive hydrocephalus may be controlled with a shunt. Cysts in the spinal canal can sometimes be excised.

Trypanosomiasis. African sleeping sickness may be manifest as an acute encephalopathy in the third or fourth week of the illness. There may be Parkinsonian features, but localising signs are rare. Sometimes there are features of meningitis and the spinal fluid shows pleocytosis with trypanosomes.

The systemic disease is usually treated with antrypol 1 g i.v. weekly for 10 weeks or combined with tryparsamide 30 mg/kg in 10 ml of water intravenously. When the nervous system is involved melarsen oxide 3·5 mg/kg for four days is advised and the course may be repeated after two weeks. These drugs are toxic to nerve tissue and skin. In Chagas disease there is no satisfactory therapy.

Schistosomiasis. Involvement of the brain and spinal cord are associated particularly with *Schistosoma mansoni* infestation. An acute or subacute encephalopathy may develop or, occasionally, an expanding granuloma. Paraplegia may be caused from granuloma with compression or myelopathy. Ova are usually present in faeces (*S. mansoni*) or urine (*S. haematobium*) and the spinal fluid shows lymphocytosis. Eosinophilia is common.

Treatment usually consists of niridazole by mouth 25 mg/kg daily (in two doses) for 10 days or stibocaptate 6 to 10 mg/kg i.m. weekly for 5 weeks.

Filariasis. The filarial diseases show a circumscribed geographical distribution and are common in West Africa. *Filaria loa loa* and *Wuchereria bancrofti* are spread by mosquitoes and produce fever, localised swelling at the site of the bite due to allergic reaction, and, occasionally, encephalitis. The *loa loa* is sometimes seen under the conjuctiva and microfilaria can be identified in blood. Eosinophilia is common. Onchocerciasis is spread by the buffalo gnat and causes skin disease and blindness. The organism is found in cutaneous nodules (onchus) and skin.

Diethylcarbamazepine is the drug of choice and kills microfilaria of all species. The dose is 2 mg/kg three times daily by mouth for three weeks. If the eye is involved in onchocerciasis a smaller initial dose is advisable. Antihistamines and corticosteroids applied topically to the eye are useful in controlling reactions.

20

Metabolic Disorders

The management of encephalopathy due to metabolic causes frequently falls within the realm of the general physician. It is unusual for the neurologist to be involved in the long-term management of uraemia or hepatic encephalopathy. Nevertheless, a variety of metabolic disorders may need to be considered in the differential diagnosis of coma of unknown cause, and some knowledge of the immediate management of these conditions is necessary. Specific disorders such as Wilson's disease lead to a well-defined clinical picture and require considerable expertise in their long-term management. Some aspects of endocrine disease have already been covered under muscle diseases, and this chapter concentrates on metabolic and endocrine causes of encephalopathy, electrolyte disturbance, vitamin deficiency, and exogenous poisoning, including drug overdose and addiction.

HEPATIC AND RENAL FAILURE

Hepatic Encephalopathy. This is most often seen after portocaval anastomosis and may be precipitated by gastrointestinal haemorrhage. It is also seen in acute hepatitis and in the end stage of cirrhosis.

Coma may develop rapidly and in milder cases the signs fluctuate. It may be preceded by flapping tremor, thought disorders, changes of affect and a variety of other focal neurological signs, involving motor systems and higher neurological functions. Hepatic fetor is characteristic and constant. The EEG shows a diffuse excess of slow activity and, in some instances, triphasic delta waves. There is a good correlation between EEG changes and clinical progress. A basal ganglia disorder with choreoathetotic movements may occur. A chronic spastic paraplegia is occasionally seen with massive portocaval shunting.

The basic treatment consists of withdrawal of protein from the diet. Nutrition is provided by 20 per cent dextrose via a gastric tube giving 1600 Cal. daily or 20 per cent dextrose into a large vein. The bacterial content of the gut should be altered by administration of neomycin. The initial dosage may need to be as high as from 6 to 12 g a day with a maintenance dose of 1 g four times a day. Only a small percentage of neomycin is absorbed.

Lactulose is valuable in producing rapid emptying of the gut and reducing the colonic pH. A large dose of 100 g per day may be initially required with a maintenance dose of between 40 and 60 g a day. This disaccharide is given in a 50 per cent solution.

When there is an improvement protein is cautiously reintroduced by 20 g increments on alternate days. Patients with chronic hepatic failure need to be maintained on 40 to 50 g of protein daily. Occasionally, surgical exclusion of the colon is advised if there is difficulty in eliminating protein-forming organisms.

It has now been shown that levodopa has an arousal effect in patients with hepatic coma. The administration of levodopa 1·5 to 2 g daily may assist in alerting the patient although there is no evidence that it has any effect on the long-term prognosis.

The prognosis in hepatic coma is poor unless bleeding, alcohol, drugs or infection have precipitated failure.

Renal Failure. Renal failure may lead to myoclonus, convulsions and coma. The blood urea is raised. In chronic cases there is often anaemia and hypertension. Renal dialysis may be needed in the acute case as well as treatment of the cause. In chronic renal failure maintenance dialysis and transplantation are used in selective cases.

An acute cerebral disturbance characterised by headache, vomiting, and a slowing in the EEG may develop a few hours after the start of dialysis. The blood urea is usually very high and the problem arises because of slow urea transport over the blood brain barrier, resulting in cerebral oedema. A dialysing solution containing 140 mmol of sodium per litre should be used. Chronic dialysis dementia is discussed on page 109.

The peripheral neuropathy associated with uraemia responds to dialysis although there may be a delay of some months before it happens. Renal transplantation leads to gradual improvement.

ENDROCRINE DISORDERS

THYROID DISEASE

Myxoedema. The muscle complications have been referred to in Chapter 18. Dementia, coma, and ataxia due to thyroid insufficiency are the other important central neurological complications. A bilateral carpal tunnel syndrome may be associated with myxoedema.

The dementia comes on insidiously and may go unrecognised unless the classical features of the disease are sought. There may be an organic psychosis. All patients with a presenile dementia should have thyroid function studies. The condition is reversible by giving thyroxine up to 200 μg daily. The dose should be built up gradually, starting with 50 μg daily.

Myxoedema coma is very rare as a spontaneous development. It usually develops in the cold and malnourished and this is a medical emergency. Tri-iodothyronine is the preparation of choice in myxoedema coma. An initial dose of 5 μg daily by intramuscular injection is gradually increased each day up to 20 μg. Even with great care there is a mortality of 50 per cent. If cardiac failure does not occur the drug can be continued by mouth or, alternatively, 100 μg of thyroxine. Many patients with myxoedema coma have hypothermia; they are slowly warmed in a warm room and with adequate blankets. It is necessary to give corticosteroids in myxoedema coma during the critical stage, and hydrocortisone 50 to 100 mg intravenously should be given until consciousness is regained and the body temperature returns to normal. The dose of hydrocortisone should then be gradually tailed off.

The cerebellar ataxia associated with myxoedema often escapes detection and the diagnosis should be considered in any patient with ataxia of obscure origin. The condition responds to treatment with thyroxine. Recovery takes place over approximately two months but occasionally the disability is permanent.

Cretinism. Treatment fails unless the diagnosis is made early. If therapy starts in the neonatal period there is normal development. Some variation in response will still depend on the age in fetal life when deficiency developed. The dose required is larger than might be expected. A starting dose of 100 μg of thyroxine should be increased to 200 μg by the age of two.

Hyperthyroidism. The central effects include choreoathetosis which resolves when the condition is treated. In a thyroid storm there is confusion and excitability. Propranolol 40 mg t.d.s. is helpful in reducing the tachycardia. Up to 5 mg intravenously is given in an acute crisis. Chlorpromazine 50 to 100 mg six-hourly is used for sedation. Myopathy is discussed on page 214.

ADDISON'S DISEASE

Patients with chronic Addison's disease have a low blood pressure, excessive melanin pigmentation, muscle weakness, and lethargy. In an acute crisis there may be mental confusion, convulsions and coma. Circulatory collapse is common. An acute adrenal crisis often follows the sudden cessation of large doses of corticosteroids.

In acute failure, hydrocortisone 100 mg every eight hours should be administered with a loading dose of 300 mg. The hydrocortisone should be given in an infusion of isotonic saline. The amount required will vary, but 3 litres a day is an average requirement. On recovery, the hydrocortisone should be given in a dose of 25 mg intramuscularly six-hourly while the patient resumes oral feeding. The overall situation must then be fully assessed.

Maintenance therapy consists of 25 to 37·5 mg of cortisone acetate daily. It is common to divide the dose and give 25 mg in the morning and 12·5 mg at night. Fludrocortisone 0·1 to 0·3 mg daily may be required as a mineralocorticoid.

Adrenal failure may be due to metastatic tumours from bronchial carcinoma and the patient often has evidence of cerebral metastases.

DIABETES MELLITUS

Ketotic Diabetic Coma. This may be the presenting feature of diabetes, especially in children, or in inadequately treated or brittle diabetics. The main emphasis in management is restoring fluid balance and reducing the blood sugar to normal levels. Large amounts of fluid are required to correct dehydration. Four to six litres of water together with 400 to 600 mmol of sodium and 200 to 400 mmol of potassium may be required.

It has been customary to administer crystalline insulin in large doses subcutaneously and intravenously. The dosage required varies but may be in the region of 200 units in the first 24 hours. The regime described by Alberti, using small frequent doses of insulin, is becoming increasingly widely used and has been found to be an easier and effective way of managing diabetic coma. Ten units intravenously and ten units intramuscularly are given initially, followed by five units intramuscularly hourly until the blood sugar is at a satisfactory level. If a large dose regime is to be used, 50 units intravenously with a similar amount subcutaneously is suitable.

Four to eight litres of fluid will be required in the first 24 hours. Isotonic saline should be given immediately and it is reasonable to add up to 15 mmol of potassium to each litre. Hypotonic saline is of value in older patients and careful monitoring of central venous pressure is necessary. Bicarbonate is not indicated as a routine. Isotonic saline may be replaced by 5 per cent dextrose saline once the blood glucose level is in the region of 11 mmol/litre.

Once the treatment of diabetic coma is under control, the reason for the coma should be sought. An underlying infection may be responsible and this may sometimes have caused diarrhoea and vomiting. When coma has been treated the patient will require restabilisation on an appropriate insulin compound.

Non-Ketotic Diabetic Coma. In this condition the blood glucose rises from 50 to 60 mmol/litre or higher in the absence of ketoacidosis. There is severe dehydration with a secondary hypernatraemia. Serum osmolality should range between 285 and 295 mOsm/kg. In non-ketotic coma the serum osmolality may be 375 mOsm/kg. The treatment of this condition is with the administration of hypotonic saline and insulin. The dose of insulin required may be as little as 30 to 50 units. The reason for non-ketotic coma in diabetics is obscure but such patients may do well after recovery, requiring only a small dose of insulin. The prognosis is poor unless immediate treatment is undertaken.

There may be other hypo-osmolar states without diabetes mellitus being present. The most important causes are severe diarrhoea, diabetes insipidus, and incorrect administration of electrolyte solutions.

HYPOGLYCAEMIA

The most important cause of hypoglycaemia is treated diabetes mellitus. Hypoglycaemia is common in the early stages of control of diabetes and is particularly likely in brittle diabetics. It is an important complication of long-acting insulin preparations, and certain hypoglycaemic agents, for example, chlorpropamide. In children, hypoglycaemia must always be considered as a possible cause of fits. A blood sugar estimation is essential in any child presenting with a seizure. Leucine hypersensitivity and other non-diabetic causes may be responsible in childhood. Insulin-secreting tumours of the pancreas are a rare cause of hypoglycaemia and present considerable diagnostic difficulties. The symptoms of hypoglycaemia in diabetes consists of light-headedness, vertigo, sweating, and altered mental behaviour. If the condition is untreated there is coma, and fits may be a further complication. In anyone presenting in coma, 10 to 40 g of 50 per cent intravenous glucose should be given. An alternative is 1 to 10 units of intramuscular glucagon.

An insulin-secreting tumour of the pancreas should be considered in anyone presenting with atypical fits. Such seizures may be preceded by diplopia and abnormal mental behaviour, and are unusually prolonged. Unfortunately, if the diagnosis is not made, there may be irreversible brain damage eventually. In all instances a fasting blood glucose or blood sugar obtained during an attack, will indicate hypoglycaemia. A prolonged fast will be necessary for serial blood glucose estimations combined with blood insulin levels. A high blood insulin level in relation to the blood glucose is the most important diagnostic indicator of an islet cell tumour. The diagnosis is eventually confirmed by laparotomy and direct inspection of the pancreas. Single or multiple adenomata may be present and on occasions islet cell hyperplasia is the cause of excess insulin secretion. Surgical resection of the adenoma or partial pancreatectomy is necessary.

DYSCALCAEMIA

Parathyroid Disease—Hypercalcaemia. This may be due to primary hyperparathyroidism, vitamin D excess, carcinoma, myelomatosis, sarcoidosis, thyrotoxicosis and the milk-alkali syndrome. If the rise is acute, there is headache, vomiting and, in extreme cases, mental confusion, coma and sudden death. Severe hypercalcaemia causes damage to the renal tubules.

Corticosteroids in the form of prednisolone reduce the level of serum calcium, particularly in sarcoidosis. An oral dose of 30 to 60 mg of prednisolone a day is necessary and the response is slow, taking as long as two weeks. Sodium sulphate infused as 2 litres over nine to twelve hours promotes calcium excretion. Disodium edetate is an effective chelating agent in acute hypercalcaemia. This is dissolved in 500 ml of normal saline and given in a dose of 15 mg/kg body weight over four hours. Sodium phosphate may be infused in an intravenous solution containing a mixture of Na_2HPO_4 and KH_2PO_4. It is not recommended because extracellular precipitation of calcium is common.

Calcitonin is a recent advance in treating hypercalcaemia. It may be valuable in a crisis. A single dose will reduce the calcium level for six hours. One hundred MRC units (salmon) subcutaneously is the recommended dose. It should not be used other than in an acute crisis.

Mithramycin has been shown to lower the serum calcium in malignant disease. The drug is a cytotoxic antibiotic and reduces the level of serum calcium within 24 hours of administration. The dose is 25 μg/kg daily. It should only be given for 3 days at a time followed by an interval of 7 to 10 days.

Hypocalcaemia. The most important causes are primary hypoparathyroidism, hypoparathyroidism following thyroidectomy, rickets, malabsorption, renal failure, and anticonvulsant therapy. Acute hypocalcaemia causes raised intracranial pressure, convulsions and tetany. This is best relieved by calcium gluconate 10 ml of a 10 per cent solution intravenously. Oral dihydrotachysterol 1·25 mg to 3·75 mg t.d.s. may be added as the effect of calcium gluconate is short-lived. When calcium appears in the urine the dose must be adjusted to achieve normal serum calcium levels.

Primary idiopathic hypoparathyroidism may cause mental retardation and epilepsy. Intracranial calcification occurs. The treatment is with dihydrotachysterol 1·25 mg daily or calciferol 1·25 to 5 mg daily. Regular checks should be kept on blood and urinary calcium. Primary hypoparathyroidism usually occurs under the age of sixteen and recovery of the neurological deficits may be incomplete.

ELECTROLYTE DISTURBANCES

Hypokalaemia and Hyperkalaemia. Potassium deficiency may be due to inadequate intake or excessive loss from the gastrointestinal tract and kidneys. The clinical features of hypokalaemia are muscle weakness, paralytic ileus, and myocardial abnormalities including an increased sensitivity to digitalis. The effect on muscle is to cause changes in membrane potential. The various forms of periodic paralysis have been described in Chapter 18. Potassium depletion should be corrected cautiously and 20 mmol of potassium chloride given intravenously per hour is the maximum level of replacement. It is difficult to measure the exact amount of total body deficiency and very rapid administration of large quantities will be cardiotoxic.

Hyperkalaemia may be caused by rapid administration of potassium with or without renal failure. Calcium gluconate in a 10 per cent solution will counteract the ill effect of potassium on the heart. Fifty ml of 10 per cent solution may be given intravenously.

Water and Sodium Metabolism. As sodium is the principal extracellular cation it is closely bound with extracellular fluid volume. Sodium and water may be lost in isotonic amounts, usually from the gastrointestinal tract. Water is lost in excess of sodium after prolonged exposure to the sun or because of inadequate fluid intake. Diabetes mellitus and diabetes insipidus are other causes. Sodium may be depleted in excess of water when fluid replacement therapy is sodium deficient. There is, also, sodium loss in Addison's disease and renal failure. All the above situations cause a contraction of the extracellular volume.

There is extracellular fluid expansion in water intoxication. Obsessive-compulsive water-drinking is an important cause of this. Inappropriate secretion of antidiuretic hormone, which may be associated with carcinoma, also causes expansion of the extracellular volume.

In severe isotonic fluid loss there is circulatory collapse and eventual coma. Severe hyponatraemia leads to fatigue, apathy, and muscle weakness. Water loss in extreme circumstances will lead to mental deterioration, hallucinations, and coma. Water intoxication also causes an encephalopathy with mental confusion and seizures.

Salt and water loss should be corrected with isotonic saline. In severe cases the first litre may need to be infused over ten minutes. Isotonic saline will correct mild hyponatraemia or hypernatraemia if renal function is normal. Severe changes in osmolality have an adverse effect on the brain. In hyponatraemia it may be necessary to give 500 mmol to raise a sodium level from 120 to 130 mmol/litre. In hypernatraemia, 4 to 6 litres of additional water may be required to reduce the sodium concentration to safe levels.

Hypomagnesaemia. This may be caused by loss from the gut or following prolonged parenteral feeding without correct supplements. Haemodialysis and renal tubular damage are other causes. Magnesium deficiency causes muscle weakness, psychotic behaviour, and fits. Pure magnesium deficiency is rare. The deficiency should be corrected with parenteral fluids containing magnesium chloride.

INBORN ERRORS OF METABOLISM

Porphyria. Acute intermittent porphyria is the type most commonly associated with neurological disturbance. The presenting feature is recurrent abdominal pain. The commonest objective neurological disturbance is a severe motor neuropathy with autonomic involvement. An encephalopathy with fits and eventual coma occurs. The neurological complications are usually precipitated by a drug that affects porphyrin metabolism. The most important are barbiturates, sulphonamides, oral contraceptives, methyldopa, oral hypoglycaemic agents, and chlordiazepoxide. The correct management is to make the diagnosis at an early stage by detecting increased porphobilinogen in the urine. Precipitating factors of neurological disease are then avoided.

The severe neuropathy of porphyria may require respirator care. When there is a severe tachycardia, propranolol 40 mg three times daily is helpful.

The variegate type of porphyria is associated with similar neurological problems but this is rarer.

Phenylketonuria. This is an autosomal recessive disorder with a deficiency of phenylalanine hydroxylase. Failure to recognise the disease in infancy results in mental retardation and epilepsy. The diagnosis is made by routine screening for plasma phenylalanine levels, using a flurometric technique. The ferric chloride test is a less reliable but simple test using urine.

Treatment consists of reducing the phenylalanine content of the diet to 50 mg/kg/day for three years. This is achieved by feeding on aminoacid mixture with phenylalanine supplements. After this time the requirement falls to 20 mg/kg/day.

Homocystinura. The disease presents with mental retardation, thromboembolism and skeletal abnormalities. The plasma methionine is raised. The treatment is dietary restriction of methionine with adequate cystine.

WILSON'S DISEASE

This inborn error of copper metabolism is inherited as an autosomal recessive. The serum concentration of caeruloplasmin is reduced. Copper is deposited in the tissues and, in particular, the liver and brain. There is increased excretion of copper in the urine which may cause secondary renal damage.

Wilson's disease may present either with cirrhosis of the liver or with involvement of the central nervous system, including an abnormal mental state and involuntary movements. The Kayser-Fleischer ring found in the cornea is diagnostic but may only be seen with the slit lamp.

The drug choice in the treatment of this disease is D-penicillamine, a chelating agent that promotes excretion of copper in the urine. The dose of D-penicillamine is 500 mg three times daily and this has to be given for life. It may cause acute skin reactions, fever, lymphadenopathy, leucopenia, thrombocytopenia, and a nephrotic syndrome. An alternative drug is triethylenetetramine dihydrochloride in a dose of 400 mg three times daily. The prognosis is favourable in cases diagnosed early.

ALCOHOLISM

There is no simple definition of alcoholism. However, most alcoholics show an increasing tolerance and physical dependence on the drug. Withdrawal of ethyl alcohol is associated with pronounced physical and mental symptoms. In addition, the chronic alcoholic suffers from established physical disease in the form of cirrhosis of the liver and a variety of neurological disturbances, although some of these physical problems improve after prolonged abstinence.

Alcohol Withdrawal. The sudden cessation of alcohol in someone accustomed to sustained high blood levels results in tremulousness, convulsions, and delirium tremens. In the early stage of withdrawal, sweating and vomiting may predominate. Within 48 hours the patient is hallucinated and may have seizures. There is a rebound increase in rapid eye movement sleep. There may eventually be disorientation, exhaustion, hyperthermia and circulatory collapse. The patient may die in the state of acute withdrawal or recover spontaneously over several days.

The principles involved in managing controlled withdrawal of alcohol are common to other forms of addiction such as barbiturates, amphetamine, and opium derivatives. Some patients have defined psychiatric problems that are relevant to the addictive process and must be assessed. The general health of the individual must be evaluated and special care taken in the presence of chronic physical disease such as angina pectoris or asthma. Apart from specific measures taken to control the withdrawal symptoms, vitamin deficiencies must be corrected, and dehydration which may follow excessive vomiting. The most effective drug in controlling withdrawal symptoms is chlordiazepoxide (Librium). Very large doses are required and 300 to 500 mg/day may be needed in the initial stages. The dose is subsequently reduced by daily assessment but the drug should be continued for several weeks at least and at a dose range of 60 to 90 mg daily. An alternative is paraldehyde 40 to 80 ml daily but it is less acceptable because of its smell and difficulty of administration.

Alcoholic Peripheral Neuropathy. This is a nutritional disorder due to a deficiency of thiamine. A poor appetite together with a large alcohol intake causes a mixed motor and sensory neuropathy. In severe cases that are diagnosed late, recovery is slow. Thiamine 100 mg intravenously for five days followed by 10 to 15 mg orally is the appropriate treatment, but full recovery may not take place for many months and may not be complete.

Wernicke's Encephalopathy. This is a serious complication of thiamine deficiency in the alcoholic and is associated with eye movement disorders, ataxia, and Korsakoff's psychosis. The changes are permanent unless the condition is treated rapidly with parenteral thiamine in a minimum dose of 100 mg intravenously until clinical recovery is apparent. Care must be taken to avoid giving large quantities of parenteral glucose which will reduce available thiamine.

Alcoholic Ataxia and Dementia. Chronic cerebellar ataxia in isolation or associated with a progressing dementia occur in chronic alcoholism. The role of thiamine deficiency in these states is dubious. They probably result from the direct toxic effect of alcohol on cerebellar and cortical neurones. Treatment with thiamine or other vitamins is disappointing. Sometimes if the patient abstains for a prolonged period of time there is some spontaneous improvement.

VITAMIN DEFICIENCIES

Vitamin B12 (cyanocobalamin). The vitamin is absorbed in the terminal ileum. The classical cause is due to lack of gastric intrinsic factor, but Crohn's disease, diphylobothrium latum infestation, tropical sprue, and postgastrectomy states may all cause deficiency.

There may be peripheral neuropathy, subacute combined myelopathy, optic neuropathy and dementia. The typical neurological picture begins with paraesthesia in the feet and hands followed by clumsiness and weakness of the arms and legs. There is evidence of involvement of the motor pathways in the spinal cord. The ankle jerks are usually absent but the plantar responses extensor. The diagnosis is confirmed with a serum B12 level under 100 ng/litre.

Treatment consits of replacing the vitamin deficiency with regular injections of hydroxycobalamin for life, except when the cause of the deficiency is remediable. An initial dose of 1 mg intramuscularly is given. It is customary to give larger doses than are necessary. Maintenance on 1 mg a month is satisfactory.

Vitamin B1 (thiamine). Peripheral neuropathy (dry beriberi) and Wernicke's encephalopathy are the neurological disturbances associated with thiamine deficiency. Inadequate dietary intake and alcoholism are the most important precipitating factors. There are no major body stores of thiamine and deficiency may develop rapidly. The daily requirement is about 0·4 mg/1000 Cal. Deficiency is corrected by 100 mg of thiamine given intravenously daily. Oral therapy can then be maintained at 10 to 15 mg daily.

Vitamin B2 (nicotinic acid). Pellagrous dementia with evidence of involvement of the skin and alimentary tract responds to nicotinamide 160 mg three times daily intravenously. Oral maintenance of 30 mg nicotinamide daily is adequate. Pellagra and beriberi may co-exist. The usual cause of nicotinamide deficiency is dietary deficiency or malabsorption. Nicotinamide may be formed from dietary tryptophan but simple nicotinamide replacement is the treatment of choice.

Vitamin B6 (pyridoxine). Pyridoxine deficiency causes seizures in infancy. A peripheral neuropathy and optic neuritis also occurs. The peripheral neuropathy may result from the use of isoniazid in tuberculosis (page 221). The daily requirement is 2 mg. Adequate treatment of deficiency is 150 mg daily by mouth. In infantile seizures of obscure origin, a therapeutic trial of pyridoxine is justified.

EXOGENOUS POISONING

Lead. The neurological manifestations are a neuropathy and encephalopathy. Consumption of contaminated water or inhalation of fumes are two important sources of poisoning. Children may eat paint or other lead-containing articles. Lead encephalopathy is found mainly in children, whereas the neuropathy is an adult disorder.

The treatment consists of removal of the lead source and establishment of an adequate urinary flow. In severe cases a combination of dimercaprol and sodium calcium edetate injections are given. Initially, dimercaprol is given in a dose of 4 mg/kg body weight for children and 2·5 mg/kg body weight for adults. Dimercaprol is available in 2 ml ampoules in arachis oil with benzyl benzoate, each ampoule containing 100 mg. Injections are given four-hourly on the first day. The dose is reduced to six- and eight-hourly administration on the second and third days. It can then usually be stopped. Sodium calcium edetate may be started after the first injection of dimercaprol. The maximum dose is 40 mg/kg body weight. It is given daily over 12 hours in dilute solution intravenously for five days. A smaller dose of 8 mg/kg in adults and 12·5 mg/kg in children suffices in less severe cases. The dose of sodium edetate may be repeated after two to three weeks.

In severe cases of lead poisoning in children the administration of edetate may be followed by penicillamine 40 mg/kg daily for three months.

Mercury. Chronic mercury poisoning results from exposure to large amounts of vapour in laboratories or industry. The neurological manifestations of anxiety, altered affect and tremor may resolve spontaneously with removal from the mercury source. In acute intoxication dimercaprol is an effective chelating agent as 6 mg/kg body weight twice daily for ten days. Penicillamine is the other drug of value.

Arsenic. Poisoning with inorganic arsenic produces a peripheral neuropathy. Occasionally, there is spinal cord involvement as well. Tryparsamide, one of the main treatments for trypanosomiasis, causes visual failure.

An encephalopathy is induced by the intake of large quantities of trivalent organic chemicals. Multiple lesions of a vascular nature occur in the central nervous system.

Dimercaprol 4 to 5 mg/kg body weight is given intramuscularly four-hourly for 24 hours. The duration and frequency of dose has to be judged according to severity but is similar to lead poisoning.

Gold. Intoxication with gold may, occasionally, cause an encephalitis or peripheral neuropathy. These are rare and normally seen only when the side effects, which may ensue with the therapeutic use of gold, have been ignored. Regular checks should be kept on the urine, skin, blood, and mucous membranes. In severe intoxication dimercaprol or penicillamine should be used.

Carbon Monoxide. This is a colourless gas present in exhaust fumes of internal combustion engines and in many heating gases. It is not present in natural gas. It has been a common form of suicide attempt and its ill effects are due to anoxia. Carboxyhaemoglobin, which does not carry oxygen, is formed. Haemoglobin has a much greater affinity for carbon monoxide than oxygen. Exposure to 0·05 per cent carbon monoxide in inspired air for one hour will produce a 20 per cent concentration of carboxyhaemoglobin in the blood. At a concentration of 30 to 50 per cent there is headache and mental confusion. Higher levels result in coma and death. The cherry-red colour of the skin and mucous membranes is the most characteristic clinical feature. Treatment consists of ventilation with high oxygen tensions, including hyperbaric oxygen if available. Oxygen dissolved in the plasma will aid recovery of tissue anoxia. If recovery is incomplete, Parkinsonism, dementia and an organic psychosis may be permanent features.

THE NEUROTOXIC EFFECTS OF DRUGS

The number of drugs used in neurological medicine is steadily increasing. Many of the side effects that may occur with therapeutic doses have already been mentioned. The additional problem is the effect of massive overdosage or addiction which may require urgent measures. The drugs covered are those commonly used in neurological practice and no attempt is made to cover the entire therapeutic field.

CORTICOSTEROIDS

These hormones are widely used in neurological practice. Frequently, their prescription is on an empirical basis and sound scientific evidence for their value is lacking in many instances. Dexamethasone is clearly established as the drug of choice for treating cerebral oedema. The choice of steroid for use in the acute relapse of multiple sclerosis is purely arbitrary. Tradition favours ACTH or the synthetic compound tetracosactrin. However, the latter has recently been reported to induce anaphylactic shock on rare occasions and self-administration should be avoided. We are now moving towards using higher doses of oral corticosteroids or large doses of methylprednisolone over short periods of time (*see* Chapter 11).

Gastrointestinal haemorrhage and perforation may occur without a previous history of dyspepsia, and steroid administration is one of the causes of a giant gastric ulcer. There is a modification of tissue reactions and the ability of the skin to withstand trauma. Infection may spread rapidly and yet the clinical manifestations be suppressed. A serious steroid psychosis may develop unpredictably. This is common in those with a previous psychiatric history but may occur de novo. The patient is often euphoric with heightened sensory awareness but depression and suicide may follow. Hospitalisation in a psychiatric unit is required and the condition may not resolve for several months. Whatever steroid is used, the reason for using it must be carefully justified. Osteoporosis with crush vertebrae fractures are all too common in postmenopausal women. Stress fractures and aseptic necrosis of the head of the femur are seen. There is also great danger of adrenal suppression on long-term corticosteroids and it may persist for two years after stopping treatment. A boost of corticosteroids should be given to anyone who develops serious illness or who requires operation within two years of stopping long-term therapy.

ORAL CONTRACEPTIVES

These preparations contain various combinations of oestrogen and progesterone, and inhibit ovulation. The unwanted effects have been a matter of some dispute and serious consequences are rare.

There is good evidence that thromboembolic episodes may be caused and increasing belief that this tendency is reduced when the oestrogen component is low. Death may ensue from pulmonary embolism. Venous thrombosis in the limbs, cerebral venous thrombosis, and vascular disorders of the brain and retina are described. Cerebral arterial occlusion in the carotid territory may lead to hemisphere disease and hemiplegia but the vertebro-basilar circulation is relatively often involved. Co-existing diseases such as disseminated lupus erythematosus increase the risk of cerebrovascular disturbance. There is, sometimes, chorea. Papilloedema may be part of a syndrome of benign intracranial hypertension. Retrobulbar neuritis has been reported but the causal relationship is tenuous.

Migraine may be aggravated and a change in the clinical pattern to show focal features may precede a cerebrovascular episode. It should therefore be regarded as a warning signal and a reason for stopping the therapy. Epilepsy may also be aggravated (Bickerstaff 1975).

Drugs that stimulate enzyme induction in the liver such as phenytoin may increase the rate of metabolic turnover of oestrogen and progesterone and so diminish the contraceptive effect.

ANTIMICROBIAL AGENTS

Penicillins. The important side effect on the nervous system is the injection of excessive amounts intrathecally and into the ventricular system. Only 20 000 units (12 mg) should be injected intrathecally. Large doses produce arachnoiditis, convulsions, and coma. Very large doses of intravenous penicillin may produce convulsions. The inadvertent injection of penicillin into a sciatic nerve produces severe pain and loss of function. Recovery may be incomplete.

ANTICONVULSANTS

The toxic effects resulting from treatment of epilepsy have already been described. However, overdosage may result in more serious consequences in some of the drugs used.

Phenytoin. Intravenous overdosage of the drug causes cardiovascular collapse and central nervous system depression. Acute overdosage causes gross ataxia, vertigo, confusion and hallucinations. There is no specific antidote. Chronic toxic effects include a cerebellar syndrome, gingival hyperplasia, osteomalacia, peripheral neuropathy, hirsutism, and megaloblastic anaemia. Phenytoin is much less likely to cause such toxic effects if the plasma level is kept between 10 and 20 mg/litre.

Barbiturates. Phenobarbitone as a treatment for epilepsy is the only reasonable indication for barbiturate usage in neurological practice. Chronic overdosage with phenobarbitone causes nystagmus, unsteadiness, drowsiness, depression, and impotence. Hyperactivity may be produced in children. Massive overdosage is worse with a short or medium acting barbiturate. The EEG may remain flat for several days. General supportive measures are given but a forced diuresis using mannitol may be tried.

Barbiturates are now widely used by drug abusers. Barbiturate addiction is often mixed with opioid and alcohol dependence. Intoxication is similar to that with alcohol. The victim is slow and paranoid, with faulty judgement. He shows nystagmus and is often ataxic. Withdrawal causes weakness, tremulousness, and convulsions. Sudden cessation of barbiturates in patients on large doses may cause death. It is recommended that the short-acting pentobarbitone should be substituted to a level of slight toxicity over one day and then gradually reduced. Withdrawal takes at least two weeks.

Benzodiazepines. This group of drugs is widely used for the treatment of anxiety and insomnia as well as epilepsy. The main side effects are cardiac and respiratory depression when diazepam and clonazepam are used intravenously. In susceptible individuals, even small doses cause drowsiness. The drugs are safe. Massive overdosage of 600 mg of diazepam may not cause death. The treatment of overdosage is supportive measures for the blood pressure and respiration. Spontaneous complete recovery will occur.

Suxinamides. On the whole, suxinamides are well tolerated. There may be gastrointestinal upset, nausea, vertigo, and drowsiness, and rarely a Parkinsonian picture has been reported. Massive overdosage has not been a problem in our experience. There is no specific antidote.

Carbamazepine. With carbamazepine there may be aplastic anaemia, thrombocytopenia purpura, skin rashes, ataxia and liver damage, and increased skin pigmentation. All these may appear on chronic dosage. Massive overdosage causes drowsiness and coma with circulatory collapse. There is no specific antidote and supportive measures must be applied.

ANTIDEPRESSANTS

Monoamine Oxidase Inhibitors. Tranylcypromine (Parnate) and phenelzine (Nardil) are the best known drugs in this group. Tranylcypromine has a greater stimulant effect than phenelzine.

An acute toxic reaction due to an overdose causes agitation, psychotic behaviour and convulsions. The temperature rises and there is marked hypotension. It is unwise to administer any additional drugs to combat the toxic state. If possible, the blood pressure should be raised by elevating the foot of the bed, and sympathomimetic agents should be avoided. The temperature is reduced by fans and sponging. Death may ensue but full recovery is common after a week under continuous hospital observation.

Monoamine oxidase inhibitors have chronic toxic effects on the liver. This is an unpredictable response. Postural hypotension is an occasional problem and, in some individuals, sweating, severe insomnia, and hallucinations.

One of the most important facets of monoamine oxidase inhibitor usage is the interaction with other drugs and foods. They delay the breakdown of sympathomimetic amines. The use of levodopa and sympathomimetic amines may increase central excitement. Hypertensive crisis is a serious side effect and induced by eating tyramine-containing foods such as cheese, broad beans and chianti wine. Subarachnoid haemorrhage may occur with the rise in blood pressure. Pentolinium 2 mg, subcutaneously, should be used to lower the blood pressure. The dose may be repeated after 15 minutes if necessary. All patients on monoamine oxidase inhibitors must carry a card stating they are on the drug and the food restrictions necessary.

Tricyclic Antidepressants. These produce a varied but usually prominent anticholinergic effect in therapeutic doses. Dry mouth, tachycardia, impaired accommodation, constipation, retention of urine and impotence are common. Postural hypotension occurs on higher doses and tremor and dyskinetic movements develop. Excess sweating is very common.

In acute overdosage the blood pressure usually falls. Coma ensues and there may be convulsions. Gastric lavage is indicated. If cardiac arrhythmias develop, intravenous lignocaine or propranolol should be given.

LITHIUM CARBONATE

This has been mentioned with reference to the treatment of manic depressive psychosis. Provided the therapeutic level is between 0·6 and 1·4 mmol/litre, unwanted effects do not often occur. However, a rapid rise in level may be as important as a chronic slight elevation of plasma lithium.

Intoxication causes polydypsia and polyuria, ataxia, mental confusion and coma. The EEG shows widespread slow activity. Muscle weakness also develops. Recovery from lithium intoxication is slow and the authors have seen muscle weakness and mental change persisting for three months and longer.

MAJOR TRANQUILLISERS

Phenothiazines. Chlorpromazine is the prototype. They are widely used in the treatment of schizophrenia and with less justification in anxiety states. Antiemetic properties make prochlorperazine useful in nausea. Three groups may be defined; the diethylaminopropyl, piperidine, and piperazine derivatives. Chlorpromazine belongs to the first group. Thioridiazine is a piperidine derivative and perphenazine fluphenazine and trifluoperazine are in the piperazine group. The latter have the greatest antipsychotic action.

Acute overdosage with phenothiazines is rare. They are used in large doses with remarkable tolerance. Overdosage may cause convulsions, involuntary movements and circulatory collapse. Supportive measures are indicated as there is no specific antidote.

There are certain idiosyncratic reactions on the liver and blood which are not dose related. There is cholestatic jaundice in approximately 2 per cent of patients on chlorpromazine. The jaundice clears on stopping the drug which should not be reintroduced. Blood dyscrasias are rare but can include a fatal agranulocytosis. Urticarial skin reactions and dermatitis are seen and increased photosensitivity may be present.

The neurological side effects of phenothiazines are common. Some, but not all, are dose related and their frequency varies with different preparations. There are Parkinsonian effects with chlorpromazine and even more frequently with perphenazine, prochlorperazine, and trifluoperazine. In some instances the Parkinsonian syndrome occurs because the drug has been used in an unnecessarily high dose. The policy of adding anti-Parkinsonian agents prophylactically is to be deprecated but they are useful when symptoms appear. Akithesia is a peculiar restlessness seen in patients on psychotopic drugs. It may be induced by phenothiazines, but tricyclic antidepressants are also responsible. The patient has to get up and walk around. It is a most distressing symptom and is relieved by reducing the medication. Acute dyskinesias are seen with choreiform facial movements, torticollis and, occasionally, oculogyric crisis. They are seen early in therapy. The picture is most dramatic and may be misdiagnosed as hysteria or even tetanus. They cease after 48 hours if the drug is stopped. Diazepam 10 mg intravenously is a valuable temporary form of relief. Tardive dyskinesia consist of choreoathetoid movements which are usually facial but may be more widespread. The elderly patient is usually the victim of these movements which may persist for years and even be made worse by stopping therapy. Tetrabenazine 25 mg three times daily or haloperidol may help but the results are disappointing. The frequency of tardive dyskinesia in the elderly emphasises the need to avoid phenothiazines unless indicated for a psychotic illness.

Butyrophenones. Haloperidol is the chief member of this group. It is used for the treatment of mania and anxiety. Pharmacologically this group of drugs is similar to the phenothiazines. There is a high incidence of extrapyramidal side effects. Overdosage with it is rare. It causes involuntary movements and drowsiness. Supportive measures should be taken as required.

DRUG ABUSE

Although not strictly within the field of neurology, drug abuse is widespread and the consequences have relevance to all physicians who prescribe such drugs and who may be faced with the complications of addiction and withdrawal.

The major drugs of abuse can be divided conveniently into several groups: opium and its derivatives, barbiturates, alcohol, sympathomimetic amines and hallucinogens. Barbiturates and alcohol have already been discussed.

Opium, Morphine and Diamorphine. If it is assumed that a person is an established addict on an opiate, the degree of tolerance developed to the drug's properties is remarkable. In a normal therapeutic environment normal doses will relieve pain for an indefinite period if given judiciously, although one must accept that in the terminal patient whether addiction develops or not is irrelevant. If the drug is used for its euphoriant effect the frequency and dosage will rapidly rise. When withdrawal symptoms develop they reach their height at 48 to 72 hours. The victim will already have sweating, restlessness, insomnia and muscle weakness, and there will be alterations in heart rate and blood pressure. Gooseflesh skin is prominent, hence the expression going 'cold turkey'. Diarrhoea, vomiting, and failure to take fluid may lead to circulatory collapse and death. These symptoms are immediately reversed by the injection of an opiate. Total withdrawal takes about one week.

In acute poisoning, there is coma, hypoventilation and pin-point pupils. The specific treatment is with naloxone 0·4 to 1·2 mg intravenously which can be repeated until respiration is adequate. Nalorphine 10 mg intravenously is an alternative. Up to 100 mg may be given if necessary.

The most satisfactory way of managing opiate withdrawal is methadone substitution. This is given instead, and gradually withdrawn. The dose has to be monitored individually and there is some discomfort; 15 to 20 mg of methadone is a usual initial substitute when withdrawal symptoms appear. With gradual reduction each day total relatively painless withdrawal is achieved in ten days.

AMPHETAMINE

The only use for this drug in clinical neurology is in treating narcolepsy. Addiction to amphetamine creates an elevation of mood, physical strength and well being. There is little need for sleep, and mental agility appears increased. Tolerance soon develops and the danger of an acute amphetamine reaction becomes a reality. In the acute toxic state hallucinations predominate and the patient scratches at the skin. In some instances the blood pressure is greatly elevated.

Once the highly excitable state of amphetamine intoxication has been reached there may be circulatory collapse with convulsions, coma, and death. The dose required to produce a fatal amphetamine toxic state varies from as little as 15 mg to 500 mg. The speed of administration is relevant.

The treatment of the toxic state is to acidify the urine with ammonium chloride. Chlorpromazine or another phenothiazine is useful in calming the patient and lowering the blood pressure.

THE HALLUCINOGENS

Lysergic acid diethylamide is the prototype of this group of drugs. A small dose of 20 μg produces cerebral effects in susceptible individuals. There are general physical symptoms of nausea, dizziness and weakness, and, after a while, complex psychic experiences. Time seems to stand still; objects appear different in shape and colour; sensory experiences are heightened, and the perception of one sense merges into that of another. Many users feel they have a greater feeling for the world around them and a new realisation of beauty and colours. However, no tangible results follow these feelings. In a 'bad trip' there are indescribable sensations and feelings; the being seems to fragment. This may be overcome by simple support but some patients enter prolonged psychotic episodes.

In conclusion, among those who abuse drugs will be a group who have definable social and psychiatric problems that have brought them to their predicament. All drug abusers should be encouraged to seek the advice of a physician expert in the field. The treatment of a single withdrawal problem is never likely to solve the basic issues involved.

References

Halpern, D. and Meelhuysen, F. E. (1967). Duration of relaxation after intramuscular neurolysis with phenol. *Journal of the American Medical Association,* **200,** 1152–1154.

House, W. F. (1964). Transtemporal bone microsurgical removal of acoustic neuroma. *Archives of Otolaryngology,* **80,** No. 6, 597–756.

Liversedge, L. A. and Maher, R. M. (1960). Use of phenol in relief of spasticity. *British Medical Journal,* **2,** 31–33.

Lorber, J. (1971). Results of treatment of myelo-meningocele: an analysis of 524 unselected cases. *Developmental Medicine and Child Neurology,* **13,** 279–303.

Maher, R. M. (1957). Neurone selection in the relief of pain. *Lancet,* **1,** 16–19.

Marsden, C. D. (1976). Advances in the management of Parkinson's disease. *Scottish Medical Journal,* **2,** 139–148.

McKenzie, I. (1965). Consequences of removing an acoustic neuroma by conventional surgical methods. *Proceedings of the Royal Society of Medicine,* **58,** 1071–1073.

Smith, H. V., Vollum, R. L., Taylor, L. M. and Taylor, K. B. (1956). The treatment of tuberculous meningitis. *Tubercle,* **37,** 301–320.

Swinburn, W. R. and Liversedge, L. A. (1973). Long-term treatment of multiple sclerosis with azathioprine. *Journal of Neurology, Neurosurgery, and Psychiatry,* **36,** 124–126.

Recommended Reading

Aird, R. B. and Woodbury, D. M. (1974). *The Management of Epilepsy*. Springfield: Thomas.

American Academy of Orthopaedic Surgeons, Committee on the care of the handicapped child (1972). *Symposium on Myelomeningocele*. St. Louis; Mosby.

Ashworth, B. (1973). *Clinical Neuro-ophthalmology*. Oxford: Blackwell.

Bickerstaff, E. R. (1975). *Neurological Complications of Oral Contraception*. Oxford: Clarendon Press.

Bradley, W. G. (1975). *Disorders of Peripheral Nerves*. Oxford: Blackwell.

Brocklehurst, G. (1976). *Spina Bifida for the Clinician*. Clinics in Developmental Medicine. London: Heinemann.

Calne, D. B. (Ed.) (1973). *Progress in the Treatment of Parkinsonism*. Advances in Neurology, Volume 3. New York: Raven Press.

Calne, D. B. (1975). *Therapeutics in Neurology*. Oxford: Blackwell.

Christie, A. B. (1974). *Infectious Diseases: epidemiology and clinical practice*, 2nd edn. Edinburgh: Churchill-Livingstone.

Consumers Association (1974). *Coping with Disablement*. London.

Critchley, M., O'Leary, J. L. and Jennett, B. (1972). *Scientific Foundations of Neurology*. London: Heinemann.

Deeley, T. J. (Ed.) (1974). *Central Nervous System Tumours*. Modern radiotherapy and oncology. London: Butterworths.

Douek, E. (1974). *The Sense of Smell and its Abnormalities*. Edinburgh: Churchill-Livingstone.

Field, J. H. (1976). *Epidemiology of Head Injuries in England and Wales*. Department of Health and Social Security. London: H.M.S.O.

Goodman, L. S. and Gilman, A. (1975). *The Pharmacological Basis of Therapeutics*, 5th edn. London: Macmillan.

Gordon, N. (1976). *Paediatric Neurology for the Clinician.* London: Spastics International Medical Publications.

Guttmann, L. (1976). *Spinal Cord Injuries: comprehensive management and research*, 2nd edn. Oxford: Blackwell.

Hall, R., Anderson, J., Smart, G. and Besser, G. M. (1974). *Fundamentals of Clinical Endocrinology*, 2nd edn. London: Pitman Medical.

Hart, F. D. (1974). *The Treatment of Chronic Pain.* London: Medical and Technical Publishing Co.

Hutchinson, E. C. and Acheson, E. J. (1975). *Strokes: natural history, pathology, and surgical treatment.* London: Saunders.

James, C. C. M. and Lassman, L. P. (1972). *Spinal Dysraphism: spina bifida occulta.* London: Butterworths.

Jennett, B. (1975). *Epilepsy After Non-missile Head Injuries*, 2nd edn. London: Heinemann.

Johnson, R. H. and Spalding, J. M. K. (1974). *Disorders of the Autonomic Nervous System.* Oxford: Blackwell.

Juel-Jensen, B. E. and MacCallum, F. O. (1972). *Herpes Simplex, Varicella, and Zoster.* London: Heinemann.

Laidlaw, J. and Richens, A. (1976). *A Textbook of Epilepsy.* Edinburgh: Churchill-Livingstone.

Licht, S. (Ed.) (1968). *Rehabilitation and Medicine:* Physical Medicine Library, Vol. 10. New Haven: Licht.

Marshall, J. (1976). *The Management of Cerebrovascular Diseases*, 3rd edn. Oxford: Blackwell.

Matthews, W. B. (Ed.) (1975). *Recent Advances in Clinical Neurology*, No. 1. Edinburgh: Churchill-Livingstone.

Mayer-Gross, Slater, E. and Roth, M. (1969). *Clinical Psychiatry*, 3rd edn. London: Ballière, Tindall, and Cassell.

McAlpine, D., Lumsden, C. E. and Acheson, E. D. (1972). *Multiple Sclerosis: a reappraisal*, 2nd edn. Edinburgh: Churchill-Livingstone.

Merskey, H. and Spear, F. G. (1967). *Pain: psychological and psychiatric aspects.* London: Ballière, Tindall, and Cassell.

Northfield, D. W. C. (1973). *The Surgery of the Central Nervous System.* Oxford: Blackwell.

Plum, F. and Posner, J. B. (1972). 2nd edn. *Diagnosis of Stupor and Coma*, 2nd edn. Philadelphia: Davis.

Potter, J. M. (1974). *The Practical Management of Head Injuries*, 3rd edn. London: Lloyd-Luke.

Ransome, J., Holden, H. and Bull, T. R. (1973). *Recent Advances in Otolaryngology, No. 4.* Edinburgh: Churchill-Livingstone.

Richens, A. (1976). *Drug Treatment of Epilepsy.* London: Kimpton.

Seddon, Sir H. (1975). *Surgical Disorders of Peripheral Nerves*, 2nd. edn. Edinburgh: Churchill-Livingstone.

Stoddart, J. C. (1976). *Intensive Therapy*. Oxford: Blackwell.

Sunderland, S. (1968). *Nerves and Nerve Injuries*. Edinburgh: Churchill-Livingstone.

Till, K. (1975). *Paediatric Neurosurgery*. Oxford: Blackwell.

Victor, M., Adams, R. D. and Collins, G. H. (1971). *The Wernicke-Korsakoff Syndrome*. Oxford: Blackwell.

Walton, J. N. (1974). *Disorders of Voluntary Muscle*, 3rd edn. Edinburgh: Churchill-Livingstone.

Walton, J. N. (1977). *Brain's Diseases of the Nervous System*, 8th edn. Oxford: Oxford University Press.

White, J. C. and Sweet, W. H. (1969). *Pain and the Neurosurgeon*. Springfield: Thomas.

Williams, D. (Ed.) (1975). *Modern Trends in Neurology—6*. London: Butterworths.

Wolff's Headache and Other Head Pain (1972). Revised by Dalessio. New York: Oxford University Press.

Appendix 1
Voluntary Organisations in the United Kingdom

Central Council for the Disabled,
34 Eccleston Square, London SW1V 1PE.
Publications—holidays—access problems for disabled.

British Council for Rehabilitation of the Disabled,
Tavistock House South, Tavistock Square, London WC1H 9LB.
Training of handicapped people—courses.

British Epilepsy Association,
3 Alfred Place, London WC1.
Improve public understanding—assist research.

Disablement Income Group,
Queens House, 180 Tottenham Court Road, London W1P OBD.
Advisory service—local branches.

Disabled Living Foundation,
346 Kensington High Street, London W14 8NS.
Publishes books about disability and aids.

Spastics Society,
12 Park Crescent, London W1N 4EQ.
Aids—booklets—support services, schools, centres.

Parkinson's Disease Society,
81 Queens Road, London SW19 8NR.
Information and advisory service.

Multiple Sclerosis Society,
4 Tachbrook Street, London SW1V 1SJ.
Voluntary welfare—local branches—supports research.

Muscular Dystrophy Group,
26 Borough High Street, London SE1 9QG.
Supportive—local branches—research.

National Fund for Research into Crippling Diseases,
Vincent House, 1 Springfield Road, Horsham. Sussex RH12 2BR.
Research—publications—equipment.

British Polio Fellowship,
Bell Close, West End Road, Ruislip, Middlesex HA4 6LP.
Welfare service—homes—holidays—sport.

Spinal Injuries Association,
24 Nutford Place, London W1H 6AN.

Friedreich's Ataxia Group,
Bolsover House, 5 Clipstone Street, London W1.
Supportive—funds research.

Disabled Drivers Association,
The Hall, Ashwellthorpe, Norwich NOR8 9W.

Disabled Drivers Motor Club,
39 Templewood, London W13 8DU
Advice about car insurance for the disabled.

Appendix 2
Financial Allowances in the United Kingdom and Other Sources of Help

The Department of Health and Social Security provides allowances and the details are given in several pamphlets such as 'Help for Handicapped People' (HB1), Pensions (NP25), and Family Benefits (FB1). The most important allowances are as follows:

Sickness Benefit—this is payable for a period of 28 weeks during illness that prevents work to those who have paid National Insurance contributions.

Industrial Injury Benefit—is paid in place of Sickness Benefit to those who have sustained an incapacitating injury at work.

Invalidity Pension—can begin after 28 weeks of illness as a continuation of sickness benefit.

An Invalidity Allowance is added to the Invalidity Pension when appropriate (pamphlet NI 210).

Attendance Allowance is payable to adults or in respect of children over two years of age who are living at home and require a lot of care and attention. It can begin when the period of incapacity reaches six months. The payment is tax-free and there are two different rates. The day rate is paid to those who do not require special care at night, and the higher (day + night) rate to those who need help throughout the 24 hours (Leaflet NI 205).

Mobility Allowance. In recent years, those who are prevented by disability from using public transport in order to travel to work have been issued with a three-wheeled vehicle, or given a grant for the use of their own car and, where appropriate, conversion to hand controls. These benefits were combined with relief of licence and insurance.

This scheme is now being replaced by a Mobility Allowance which is taxable (pamphlet NI 211).

Various other services are available and include help from Social Workers, Home Helps, Meals-on-Wheels, and the provision of appliances such as a wheelchair, zimmer frame, elbow crutches, tripod stick, and caliper supports.

There is special provision for children, the mentally ill, and the mentally handicapped (Leaflet HB1).

The Oxford Regional Health Authority publishes booklets that have been prepared at Mary Marlborough Lodge, Oxford. The titles of these include:

Communication
Wheelchair and outdoor transport
Clothing and dressing for adults
Home management
Disabled mother
Personal care
Leisure and gardening
Housing and furniture
Hoists and walking aids
The disabled child

These are available at a cost of £1·50 each (1977) from—

Equipment for the Disabled,
2 Foredown Drive,
Portslade, Sussex BN4 2BB

Appendix 3
Proprietary Drugs

The purpose of this list is to assist in the identification of proprietary drugs when the name is known. The name of the manufacturer has been omitted. The list is restricted to drugs in common use in the practice of neurological medicine and is not intended to be comprehensive. The drugs have been listed in alphabetical order by proprietary names (as used in the United Kingdom). For further information the reader is referred to the Monthly Index of Medical Specialties (MIMS).

Aldomet	methyl dopa
Amidone	methadone
Amoxyl	amoxycillin
Anafranil	clomipramine
Ansolysen	pentolinium
Arlef	flufenamic acid
Artane	benzhexol
Atromid S	clofibrate
Bactrim	co-trimoxazole
Banocide	diethyl carbamazepine
Bellergal	phenobarbitone + belladonna alkaloids + ergotamine
Benuride	pheneturide
Brocadopa	levodopa
Brufen	ibuprofen
Butazolidin	phenylbutazone
Cafergot	ergotamine
Catapres	clonidine
Celbenin	methicillin
Ceporex	cephalexin
Ceporin	cephaloridine

Cetiprin	emepronium
Chloromycetin	chloramphenicol
Cogentin	benztropine
Dalmane	flurazepam
Dantrium	dantrolene sodium
Dartalan	thiopropazate
Decadron	dexamethasone
Declinax	debrisoquine
Deseril	methysergide
Dextran	rheomacrodex
DF 118	dihydrocodeine
Diconal	dipanone + cyclizine
Dindevan	phenindione
Disipal	orphenadrine
Distalgesic	dextropropoxyphene
Dixarit	clonidine
Doloxene	dextropropoxyphene
Dopamet	methyldopa
Endoxana	cyclophosphamide
Epanutin	phenytoin
Epilim	sodium valproate
Equanil	meprobamate
Esbatal	bethanidine
Eudemine	diazoxide
Femergin	ergotamine
Fentazin	perphenazine
Flagyl	metronidazole
Fortral	pentazocine
Furadantin	nitrofurantoin
Genticin	gentamicin
Heminevrin	chlormethiazole
Hetrazan	diethyl carbamazepine
Imuran	azathioprine
Inderal	propranolol
Indocid	indomethasone
Ismelin	guanethidene
Kemadrin	procyclidine
Largactil	chlorpromazine
Larodopa	levodopa
Lasix	frusemide
Librium	chloridazepoxide
Lingraine	ergotamine

Lioresal	baclophen
Luminal	phenobarbitone
Madopar	levodopa + benserazide
Melleril	thioridiazine
Mestinon	pyridostigmine
Marevan	warfarin
Migril	ergotamine + cyclizine + caffeine
Miltown	meprobamate
Modecate	fluphenazine
Mogadon	nitrazepam
Myambutol	ethambutol
Myotonine	bethanechol
Myanesin	mephanesin
Mysoline	primidone
Mytelase	ambenonium
Naprosyn	naproxen
Nardil	phenelzine
Negram	nalidixic acid
Neomin	neomycin
Neulactil	pericyazine
Nitoman	terabenazine
Nobrium	medazepam
Optimax	L-tryptophan
Orbenin	cloxacillin
Orgraine	ergotamine
Ospolot	sulthiame
Pacitron	L-tryptophan
Panadol	paracetamol
Parnate	tranylcypromine
Parstelin	tranylcypromine + trifluoperazine
Penbritin	ampicillin
Pertofran	desipramine
Phasal	lithium carbonate
Physeptone	methadone
Pipanol	benzhexol
Ponstan	mefenamic acid
Priadel	lithium carbonate
Probanthine	propantheline
Prostigmine	neostigmine
Pyopen	carbenicillin
Septrin	co-trimoxazole
Rivotril	clonazepam

Sanomigran	pizotifen
Seranace	haloperidol
Serc	betahistidine
Sinemet	levodopa + carbidopa
Sinequan	doxepin
Sparine	promazine
Stellazine	trifluoperazine
Stemetil	prochlorperazine
Stugeron	cinnarizine
Surmontil	trimipramine
Symmetral	amantadine
Synacthen	tetracosactrin
Talpen	talampicillin
Tegratol	carbamazepine
Tofranil	impramine
Tolnate	prothipendyl
Trasicor	oxyprenolol
Tremonil	methixene
Tryptizol	amytriptyline
Ubretid	distigmine
Uticillin	carfecillin
Valium	diazepam
Welldorm	dichloralphenazone
Zarontin	ethosuximide

INDEX

Figures in bold type are main references

Abscess
brain, 225
extradural, 226
spinal epidural, 226
subdural, 226
Acetazolamide, 213
Achondroplasia, 164
Acoustic neuroma, 98, 150, 151
ACTH
for infantile spasms, 72
in MS, 115
in myasthenia, 203
unwanted effects, 251
Actinomycosis, 235
Acupuncture, 52
Addison's disease, 241
Ageusia, 93
Airway, 3
Alcohol and trigeminal neuralgia, 57
Alcoholism, 247
Alzheimer's disease, 106, 107
Amantadine, 230
in Parkinsonism, 84
in viral encephalitis, 108
Ambemonium, 202
ε-Amino caproic acid, 128
Amitriptyline
in depression, 28
in migraine, 59
Amoebiasis, 236
Amphetamine, 257
Amphotericin B, 235
Ampicillin, 219, 220
Amyotrophic lateral sclerosis, 199
Aneurysm, cerebral, 94
Anticholinergic drugs, 84, 85
Anticoagulant therapy, 133, 134
Anticonvulsant therapy, 66
Antigen, histocompatibility, 112
Antilymphocytic serum, 116
Antrypol, 237
Anxiety state, 29, 30
Appliances, **17,** 119, **124,** 125
Aqueduct stenosis, 160
Arachnoiditis, spinal, 189
Arnold-Chiari malformation, 161
Arsenic poisoning, 250
Arteriovenous malformation
cerebral, 129
spinal, 179
Arteritis, giant cell, 56, 93
Aspergillosis, 235
Aspirin, **44,** 58, 101, 133
Ataxia telangiectasia, 111
Athetosis, 89
Atropine
for bladder, 38, 122
in myasthenia, 203
Atypical facial pain, 60, 61
Auditory tests, 96, 97
Axontmesis, 197
Azathioprine
in arteritis, 56
in MS, 115
in myasthenia, 203
in polymyositis, 212

Baclophen, 120
Barbiturate
for anxiety, 29
for insomnia, 30
overdosage, 253
Barbotage, 51
Basilar invagination, 160, 161
Beclamide, 70
Bendrofluazide, 131
Benign intracranial hypertension, 147, 148
Benserazine, 83
Benzdiazepines
in epilepsy, 69, 70
overdosage, 253
Benzhexol
in Parkinsonism, 84, 85
in schizophrenia, 33
in torticollis, 89
Benztropine, 85
Betahistidine, 99
Bethanecol chloride, 38
Bethanidine, 131
Biopsy
brain, 146, 231
in motor neurone disease, 200
muscle, 211
sural nerve, 181, 182
Bladder, 34ff
atonic, 36
deafferented, 36, 42
electrical stimulation, 39
lower motor neurone, 36
in MS, 122, 123
neck resection, 39, 122
neurogenic, 39ff
Botulism, 228
Brachial plexus neuropathy, 188, 189
Brain stem failure, 142
Bromcriptine, 85
Brompton cocktail, 46
Bulbar palsy, progressive, 199

Calcitonin, 243
Calcium metabolism
hypercalcaemia, 243
hypocalcaemia, 71, 244
Calculus, 40

Caliper, 17
Caloric texts, 97, 98
Carbachol, 38, 122
Carbamazepine
  in epilepsy, 69, 74
  in MS, 118, 123
  overdosage, 254
  in trigeminal neuralgia, 57
Carbenicillin, 219, 220
Carbidopa, 83
  in intention myoclonus, 91
Carbon monoxide poisoning, 250
Cardiac arrest, 12
Carotico-cavernous fistula, 183
Carotid stenosis, 132, 133
  endarterectomy, 133
Carpal tunnel syndrome, 194, 195
Catheter
  Foley, 37
  Gibbon, 37
Catheterisation, 37, 38
Cauda equina syndrome, 189, 190
Causalgia, 53, 196
Cavernous sinus thrombosis, 183
Cephaloridine, 219, 220
Cerebellum
  haemorrhage, 130
  tumour, 151
Cerebral death, 12
Cerebral haemorrhage, 130
Cerebral infarction, 131
Cerebral oedema, 141, 147
Cerebral palsy, 165–7
Cervical spondylosis, 173, 174
Chloral hydrate, 30
Chloramphenicol
  in enterica, 228
  in meningitis, 219, 220
Chlordiazepoxide
  in alcoholism, 247
  in anxiety, 29
  in migraine, 59
  for tremor, 88
Chlormethiazole, 70
Chloroquine, 193, 236
Chlorothiazide, 213
Chlorproguanil, 236
Chlorpromazine, 46, 56, 255
  in anxiety, 30
  in head injury, 140
  in mania, 25
  overdose, 255
  in schizophrenia, 33
  in spasticity, 120
  in tetanus, 227
Chordoma, 152
Chorea, 88, 89
  Huntington, 107
Choroid plexus papilloma, 152
Cingulotomy, 56
Cinnarizine, 99
Cisternal puncture, 217
Clioquinol, 112
Clofazimine, 229
Clofibrate, 134
Clomipramine, 28
  in narcolepsy, 80
Clonazepam
  in epilepsy, 70, 72, 75
  for myoclonus, 90
Clonidine, 59
Coarctation of aorta, 128
Codeine phosphate, 45, 58
Cold, 15
Collagen disease
  neuropathy, 193, 194
  polymyositis, 211
Collar, 173
Coma, assessment, 2
Common peroneal nerve palsy, 196
Communication, 11
Compensation neurosis, 31
Contraceptive, oral, 252
Contracture, 4
Cordotomy, 49, 50
Cortical thrombophlebitis, 136, 226
Corticosteroid therapy
  in diphtheria, 228
  in dyscalcaemia, 243
  in encephalitis, 232
  in herpes zoster, 233
  in MS, 115
  in myasthenia, 202
  in polymyositis, 211
  replacement, 241
  in tuberculosis, 223
  unwanted effects, 251
Co-trimoxazole
  in enteric fever, 228
  in meningitis, 219, 220
Counselling parents, 163
Cranial polyneuritis, 186
Craniopharyngioma, 94, 155
Craniostenosis, 159
Creatine kinase
  in malignant hyperpyrexia, 213
  in muscular dystrophy, 206
Cretinism, 240
Cricopharyngeal myotomy, 201
Crocodile tears, 186
Cryptococcus, 235
Curare and myasthenia, 9
Cyanocobalamin, 106, **192,** 248
Cyclophosphamide
  in myasthenia, 203
  in polymyositis, 212
Cysticercosis, 236
Cystometrogram, 35
Cytarabine arabinoside, 230, 232
Cytomegalic virus, 234

Dandy-Walker syndrome, 160
Dantrolene, 120
Dapsone, 229
DDAVP, 155
Deafness, 20, 21, 95–101
  childhood, 98
  in MS, 118
Debrisoquin, 131

Decerebrate state, 139–40
Dementia, 103ff
  alcoholic, 248
  assessment, 103, 104
  dialysis, 109
  in MS, 124
Depression, 25–8
Desipramine, 27
  in narcolepsy, 80
Detrusor muscle, 35
Devic's disease, 112
Dexamethasone
  in MS, 115
  in progressive stroke, 135
  in status migranicus, 58
  in tumour, 147, 148
Dextroamphetamine, 80, 257
Dextropropoxyphene, **45,** 58
Diabetes mellitus, 241
  bladder, 42
  coma, 241–3
  neuropathy, 191
Dialysis dementia, 109
Diamorphine
  addiction, 257
  analgesia, 46
Diaphragm, paralysis, 6
Diastematomyelia, 162, 163
Diathermy, 15
Diazepam, 45
  in anxiety, 29
  in epilepsy, 69, 75
  in migraine, 59
  in MS, 120
  overdosage, 253
  in torticollis, 89
  for tremor, 88
Diazoxide, 131
Dichloralphenazone, 56
Dichlorphenamide, 213
Diet
  gluten-free, 116
  in hepatic encephalopathy, 238
  in MS, 116
  sunflower oil, 116
Diethylcarbamazepine, 237
Dihydrocodeine, 45, 58
Dihydroergotamine, 59
Dihydrotachysterol, 244
Dimercaprol, 249, 250
Dipanone, 45
Diphtheria, 227
Diplomyelia, 162
Dipyridamole, 133
Disodium edetate, 243
Distigmine, 38
Driving licence
  and disability, 19
  and epilepsy, 78
Drug abuse, 256ff
Drug addiction, 257
Dupuytren's contracture, 65
Dysarthria, 22, 23
Dyscalcaemic myopathy, 215
Dyskinesia, 84
Dysphasia, 20, 21
Dystrophia myotonica, 208

Eaton-Lambert syndrome, 202, 205
Edrophonium chloride, 202
Electric convulsion therapy, 28
Electrical injury, 145
Electrical stimulation, 15, 16
  of bladder, 39
  for pain, 51
Electroencephalography
  and cerebral death, 13
  epilepsy, 62–4
Embolism, 131, 132
  fat, 141
Emepronium bromide, 35, 38
Emetine, 236
Employment
  in epilepsy, 78
  in MS, 125
Encephalitis
  measles, 234
  viral, 231
Encephalocele, 159
Endotracheal intubation, 7
Enteric fever, 228
Entrapment neuropathy, 194
Ependymoma
  spinal, 177
  ventricular, 152
Ephedrine, 202
Epilepsy, 62ff
  in adults, 74–5
  in childhood, 71–3
  classification, 63
  EEG, 62–4
  and encephalitis, 232
  focal, 74, 75
  heredity, 79
  institutional care, 79
  investigation, 62–4
  late onset, 74
  neonatal, 71
  photic, 73
  social aspects, 76–80
  status, 75, 76
Ergotamine, 58
Erythromycin, 219, 229
Ethambutol, 221, 222
Ethical considerations
  malformations, 163
  turning off respirator, 13
Ethionamide, 221, 222
Ethosuximide, 72
  overdose, 254
Ethyl chloride spray, 47, 56
Exercises, 16
Exophthalmos
  pseudotumour, 182, 184
  thyroid, 182

Facial myokymia, 118
Facial pain, 60
Facial palsy, 185
  Bell's, 185

Facial palsy—*contd.*
  in herpes zoster, 185
  in MS, 118
Familial hypercholesterolaemia, 134
Familial periodic paralysis 213
Febrile convulsions, 72
Fetoscopy, 158
Filariasis, 237
Flucytosine, 236
Fludrocortisone
  in Addison's disease, 241
  in autonomic failure, 87, 111
Flufenamic acid, 45
Fluphenazine decanoate, 33, 46
Flurazepam, 30
Folate, 68, 69
Fracture
  of skull, 139
  of spine, 170
Friedreich's ataxia, 111
Fucidic acid, 233
Functional overlay, 29

Gentamicin, 233
Glaucoma
  acute, 55
  and levodopa, 84
Glioma, cerebral, 148–53
Glycerol, 135
Glycogen storage disease, 214
Gold poisoning, 250
Guanethidene, 131
Guanidine, 205
Guillain-Barré syndrome, 8, 186, 187
Gustatory sweating, 186

Haemangioblastoma
  cerebellum, 152
  vertebral body, 178, 179
Haematoma
  extradural, 130, 140, 141
  intracerebral, 141
  subdural, 106, 130, 141
Haemorrhage, intracranial, 130
Hallucinogens, 258
Haloperidol, 256
  in anxiety, 30
  for involuntary movement, 89
  in mania, 25
Head injury, 137ff
  anticonvulsants, 140
  and computerised axial tomography, 140
  cranial nerve palsies, 143
  early assessment, 137, 138
  early complications, 140–2
  early management, 138–42
  epilepsy, 144, 145
  late sequelae, 142–5
  personality change, 142
Headache, 55ff
  and cerebral tumour, 60
  and hypertension, 60
Heat therapy, 14
Hemiballismus, 89
Hemifacial spasm, 88
Heparin, 133
Hepatic encephalopathy, 238
Hepatic neuropathy, 191, 192
Herpes simplex encephalitis, 108, **231**
Herpes zoster, 233
  bladder, 42
  ophthalmicus, 56
  postherpetic neuralgia, 53
Huntington's chorea, 89, 107
Hydrocephalus, 159, 160
  normotensive, 108, 129
  shunt, 160
Hydrocortisone
  in Addison's disease, 241
  in hypothyroid coma, 240
  intrathecal, 223
  in status migranicus, 58
Hydrotherapy, 16
L-5-Hydroxytryptophane, 91
Hyperpyrexia
  and myopathy, 213
  in status epilepticus, 10
Hypertension
  control, 131
  encephalopathy, 130, 131
  headache, 60
  and Parkinsonism, 86, 87
Hyperthyroidism, 240
Hypnosis, 52
Hypochondriasis, 30
Hypoglossal-facial anastomosis, 185
Hypoglycaemia, 71, 242
Hypophysectomy, 154
Hypothermia and cerebral death, 13
Hypothyroidism, 106
Hysteria, 31, 32

Iatrogenic illness
  neuropathy, 192, 193
  psychiatric, 33
Ibuprofen, 45
Ice packs, 15
Idoxuridine, 230
  in encephalitis, 232
  in herpes zoster, 56
Imipramine, 27
  and bladder, 38
Immunosuppression in MS, 116
Incontinence of urine, 39
Indomethacin, 45, 58
Infantile spasms, 71
Infectious mononucleosis, 234
Infra-red lamp, 15
Insomnia, 30
Insulin, 241
Intensive care
  in encephalitis, 232
  monitoring, 2
  in vascular disease, 135
Intercostal neuralgia, 53, 54
Intrathecal ice cold saline, 47
Iritis, 55

Islet cell adenoma, 243
Isoniazid, 221, 222

Jakob-Creutzfeldt disease, 109, 110

Klippel-Feil syndrome, 161
Kugelberg-Welander disease, 210
Kuru, 110

Lactulose, 239
Lead poisoning, 249
Leprosy, 229
Leptospirosis, 227
Leucodystrophy
  metachromatic, 110
  multifocal, 109
Leucotomy for pain, 51
Levodopa
  cardiac arrhythmias, 84
  dyskinesia, 84
  glaucoma, 84
  in hepatic coma, 239
  in Parkinsonism, 83, 84
Lignocaine, 48
Linoleic acid, 116
Linthicum test, 97
Lithium, 25
  overdosage, 255
Lumbar puncture, 216
Lysergic acid diethylamide, 258

Macrocephaly, 159
Magnesium, 71, 245
Malaria, 235
Mania, 24, 25
Manipulation, 15
Mannitol infusion, 147
Marriage and epilepsy, 78, 79
Massage, 15
McArdle's disease, 214
Medazepam, 29
Medulloblastoma, 151
Meningioma, 94
  cerebral, 149, 150
  spinal, 177
Meningitis, 218ff
  acute, 218
  haemophilus, 220
  in leukaemia, 225
  Listeria monocytogenes, 220
  meningococcal, 218
  in neonate, 220
  pneumococcal, 220
  recurrent, 224
  in reticulosis, 225
  syphilis, 244
  tuberculous, 220, 221
Menière's disease, 98–100
Meningocele, 162
Meningomyelocele, 162
Mephanesin, 120
Meralgia paraesthetica, 47, 194
Mercaptopurine, 203
Mercury poisoning, 250
Methadone
  analgesic, 46
  in opiate addiction, 257
Methaqualone, 30
Methisazone, 230
Methyl dopa, 131
Methyl prednisolone, 49
  in MS, 115
  in myasthenia, 203
Methysergide, 59
Metoclopramide, 83
Metronidazole, 236
Migraine, 57–60
  cluster headache, 58
  and contraceptives, 60
  familial hemiplegic, 58
  ophthalmoplegic, 58
  therapy, 59
Mithramycin, 244
Monitoring
  central venous pressure, 2
  temperature, 2
Monoamine oxidase inhibitors, 26, 27
  overdosage, 254
  and tyramine, 128
Mononeuropathy, 197, 198
Morphine
  addiction, 257
  analgesic, 46, 56
Morton's metatarsalgia, 197
Motor neurone disease, 199
Multiple sclerosis, 112ff
  acute retention of urine, 40
  corticosteroid therapy, 115
  diagnosis, 112–13
  paroxysmal disorders, 123
  pregnancy, 114, 115
Muscular dystrophy
  Becker, 210
  carrier detection, 206
  Duchenne, 206
  facio-scapulo-humeral, 210
  limb girdle, 210
Myasthenia gravis, 201
  crisis, 9, 203
  neonatal, 205
Mycoses, 235
Myelography, 169, 170
Myelotomy, 50
Myoclonus
  epilepsy, 73
  intention, 12, 91
  therapy, 90, 91
Myotonia
  congenita, 209
  paramyotonia, 209
  treatment, 208
Myxoedema, 240

Nalorphine, 257
Naproxen, 45
Narcolepsy, 80

Nasopharyngeal carcinoma, 184, 185
Neostigmine, 202
Neuralgia
  glossopharyngeal, 57
  infraorbital, 47
  intercostal, 53, 54
  occipital, 47
  postherpetic, 53, 56
  trigeminal, 57, 118
Neuralgic amyotrophy, 188
Neurofibroma, spinal, 177
Neuropraxia, 197
Neurotmesis, 197
Nicotinic acid, 249
Niridazole, 237
Nitrazepam, 30, 56
  for infant spasms, 72
  for petit mal, 72
Nursing, neurological, 23

Obturator nerve palsy, 196, 197
Occupational therapy, 18ff
Olfaction, 92, 93
Onchocerciasis, 237
On/off phenomenon, 84
Ophthalmoplegia, 182–4
  exophthalmic, 214
  painful, 184
Optic neuritis, 93, 117, 118
Orbital tumour, 183
Orphenadrine, 85

Pain, 43ff
  dental, 55
  electrical stimulation for, 51
  gate theory, 43
Para-aminosalicylic acid, 221, 222
Paracetamol, 45
Paraldehyde, 75, 247
Parasympathetic system, bladder, 35
Parkinsonism, 81ff
  amantadine, 84
  carbidopa, 83
  combined therapy, 85
  and dementia, 87
  diagnosis, 82
  dopa decarboxylase inhibitor, 83
  dopamine, 82
  drug induced, 87
  drug therapy, 83–5
  hypokinesia, 82
  levodopa, 83, 84
  pathophysiology, 81
  surgical treatment, 85, 86
  tremor, 82
Penicillamine
  mercury poisoning, 250
  Wilson's disease, 247
Penicillin
  in meningitis, 219, 220
  unwanted effects, 252
Pentazocine, 45, 56
Pentolinium, 131
Perchlorperazine, 58
Pericyazine, 46, 56
Peripheral neuropathy, 186ff
Perphenazine, 46
Persistent vegetative state, 142
Personality disorder, 29ff
Pes cavus, 164
Pethidene, 46, 140
Petit mal, 72, 73
Phaeochromocytoma, 128
Phantom limb, 52, 53
Phenelzine, 27
  overdose, 254
Pheneturide, 70
Phenindione, 134
Phenobarbitone, 65, 72, 74
Phenol
  for hemifacial spasm, 88
  intrathecal, 47, 48, **121**
  perineural, 121, 122
  trigeminal, 57
Phenothiazines, 255
Phenylbutazone, 45
Phenylketonuria, 246
Phenytoin
  epilepsy, 65–9, 74, 75
  in myotonia, 208
  overdose, 253
Phobias, 30
Photic epilepsy, 73, 74
Physiotherapy, 14ff
  in MS, 116, 117
  in polymyositis, 212
Pick's disease, 106, 107
Pitressin tannate, 155
Pituitary apoplexy, 128
Pituitary tumour, 154, 155
Pizotifen, 59
Poliomyelitis, 8, 233
Polymyalgia rheumatica, 56, 212
Polymyositis, 10, 211
Polyneuropathy, acute, 8, 186
Porphyria, 245, 246
  neuropathy, 192
  respiration, 9
POSSUM, 125
Posterior column stimulation in MS, 119
Posterior interosseous neuropathy, 196
Postherpetic neuralgia, 53
Post-traumatic syndrome, 31, 145
Potassium, 4
  hyperkalaemia, 4, 244
  hypokalaemia, 244
  in periodic paralysis, 213
Pott's paraplegia, 224
Prednisolone
  in arteritis, 56
  in MS, 115
  in polymyositis, 211
Pregnancy
  and contraception, 136
  and MS, 114, 115
Primidone, 69

Probanthine, 122
Procaine amide, 209
Prochlorperazine, 99, 100
Procyclidine, 85
Progesterone in migraine, 59
Progressive muscular atrophy, 199
Proguanil, 236
Promethazine, 140
Propantheline in MS, 122
Propranolol
in hypertension, 131
in hyperthyroidism, 241
in migraine, 59
in porphyria, 246
in tremor, 88
Protamine, 133
Prothipendyl hydrochloride, 99
Psychometry, 105
Psychopathy, 31
Psychosis, organic, 32, 33
Pudenz-Heyer valve, 153
Pyrazinamide, 222
Pyridostigmine
in motor neurone disease, 200
in myasthenia, 202
Pyridoxine deficiency, 249
Pyrimethamine, 236

Quinine
in malaria, 236
in myotonia, 208

Rabies, 232, 233
Radial neuropathy, 195, 196
Radiculopathy, 186
cervical, 187
lumbar, 188
Radiotherapy, 156
Regeneration, peripheral nerve, 198
Rehabilitation, 14ff
after head injury, 138ff
after spinal injury, 170
after stroke, 135
Renal failure, 239
Renal neuropathy, 191
Respiration, assisted, 5ff
Retention of urine
acute, 37
chronic, 39
in MS, 40, 122
Rheomacrodex, 133, 135
Rhinorrhoea, cerebrospinal, 93, 224
Rhizotomy, 47, 57
Rifampicin, 221, 222
Rigidity in Parkinsonism, 82
RISA scan, 108

Schilder's disease, 112
Schistosomiasis, 237
Schizophrenia, 32, 33
and epilepsy, 32
Schuell test, 21
Scoliosis, 164
Sheepskin, 125
Shunt, ventricular, 153
Shy-Drager syndrome, 87, 110–11
Sinusitis, 55
Skin, protection of, 125
SMON, 112
Social workers, 119
Sodium, metabolism, 245
Sodium calcium edetate, 249
Sodium valproate, 69, 72
Spasticity, 119–22
Speech therapy, 19ff
Sphincter
division of, 39
external, 35
rectal, 34
Spina bifida
cystica, 161–3
occulta, 162
urinary diversion, 40
Spinal canal stenosis, 164, 190
Spinal compression, 172–8
Spinal cyst, 178
Spinal disc protrusion, 172
Spinal dysraphism, 161
Spinal fluid
in encephalitis, 225
in meningitis, 217, 218
Spinal meningioma, 177
Spinal muscular atrophy, 206
Spinal neurofibroma, 177
Spinal reticulosis, 176
Spinal shock, 37
Spinal trauma, 170–2
Spinal tumour, 176
Spiramycin, 236
Spitz-Holter valve, 153
Splints
plastic, 17
wrist, 16
Stammering, 21
Status epilepticus, 75
Steele-Richardson-Olszewski syndrome, 87
Stenosis of spinal canal, 164, 190
Stereotactic surgery
for intention tremor, 119
for pain, 50
for Parkinsonism, 86
Steroid myopathy, 214
Stibocaptate, 237
Streptomycin in tuberculous meningitis, 221, 222
intrathecal, 223
and vertigo, 102
Stroke
completed, 135–6
progressive, 135
Subacute sclerosing panencephalitis, 108, 235
Subarachnoid haemorrhage
cerebral, 128, 129
spinal, 129, 130
surgical treatment, 129
traumatic, 141

Subclavian steal syndrome, 134
Sulphadiazine, 218
Sulphinpyrazole, 101
  in transient ischaemic attack, 133
Sulthiame, 70
Suprapubic bladder drainage, 38
Suxinamides
  in epilepsy, 69
  overdose, 254
  in petit mal, 72
Sympathectomy
  for causalgia, 196
  for pain, 51
Syphilis
  cranial nerve palsies, 186
  meningitis, 224
  neuro-, 106, **228**
Syringomyelia, 163, 164

Tabes dorsalis, bladder, 42
Tarsal tunnel syndrome, 197
Tarsorrhaphy, 57, 185
Taste disorder, 92, 93
  and Bell's palsy, 185
  and head injury, 143
Temporal arteritis, 56, 93
Temporo-mandibular dysfunction, 60
Tenotomy, 207
Tensilon test, 202
Tetanus, 8, 227
Tetrabenazine, 89, 107
Tetracosactrin, *see* ACTH
Thalamotomy, stereotactic
  for MS (ataxia), 119
  for pain, 50
  for Parkinsonism, 86
  for torsion dystonia, 90
Thalidomide
  in leprosy, 229
  malformations, 164, 165
  neuropathy, 193
Thermocoagulation, trigeminal, 47
Thiamine, 248, 249
Thiethylperazine maleate, 99
Thiopentone, 75
Thiopropazate, 107
Thomsen's disease, 209
Thoracic outlet syndrome, 189
Thymectomy
  in myasthenia, 204
  in subacute sclerosing panencephalitis, 108
Thyroid myopathy, 214
Thyroxine, 240
Tic, 88
Tolosa-Hunt syndrome, 184
Torsion dystonia, 90
Torticollis, spasmodic, 89, 90
Torulosis, 235
Toxoplasmosis, 236
Tracheostomy, 6, 7
  and thymectomy, 204
Traction
  skull, 15
  spinal, 15
Tractotomy, 50
Transfer factor, 108, 116
Transient ischaemic attack, 101, 131–4
Tranylcypromine, 27
  overdose, 254
Tremor
  benign essential, 88
  Parkinsonism, 82
Tricyclic antidepressants, 27, 28
  overdosage, 225
Triethylenetetramine, 247
Trifluoperazine, 30
Trigeminal neuralgia
  idiopathic, 57
  injection, 57
  in MS, 118
  thermocoagulation, 47
Trigeminal neuropathy, 184
Trimipramine, 27
Tripod, 17
Troxidone, 69
Trypanosomiasis, 237
Tryparsamide, 237
Tuberculin, intrathecal, 223
Tuberculoma, 224
Tumour
  cerebral, 146ff
  spinal, 176

Ulnar neuropathy, 195
Ultrasound
  destruction of labyrinth, 99
  heat, 15
Urinary diversion, 39, 40

Vaccination
  complications, 234
  in MS, 117
  rabies, 232
Vascular disease, 127
  contraceptive pill, 136
  occlusive, 131–4
Venous thrombosis, cortical, 136
Vertigo, 95–102
  positional, 100, 101
Vestibular neuronitis, 100
Vibrator, electrical, 56
Visual failure, 93–5
Vitamin deficiency
  B1, 192
  B2, 192
  B6, 192
  B12, 106, **192**, 248
  D, 215
  and neuropathy, 192, 248

Walking frame, 17
Warfarin, 133
Waterhouse-Friderichsen syndrome, 218
Werdnig-Hoffman disease, 210
Wernicke's encephalopathy, 192, 248
Wheelchair, 18, 125
Wilson's disease, 82, 246
Writer's cramp, 90